The uncomfortable Confessions of a Preacher's Kid

Ronna Russell

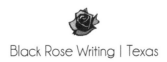

Black Rose Writing | Texas

ISBN: 978-1-68433-237-3
PUBLISHED BY BLACK ROSE WRITING
www.blackrosewriting.com

Printed in the United States of America
Suggested Retail Price (SRP) $17.95

The Uncomfortable Confessions of a Preacher's Kid is printed in Calibri
Excerpt(s) from *STILL LIFE WITH WOODPECKER* by Tom Robbins, copyright 1980 by Tom Robbins. Used by permission of Bantam Books, an imprint of Random House, a division of Penguin Random House LLC. All rights reserved.

Ronna Russell takes us on a no-holds-barred ride through her unconventional childhood and how she emerged as her own person on every level. She is fighter, a survivor, and shines a light on the things we often choose to keep in the dark. And she does it with remarkable, unapologetic honesty.

-Lisa F. Smith author of *Girl Walks Out Of a Bar*

The Uncomfortable Confessions of a Preacher's Kid is one of those stories that you couldn't make up as they say - a cascading series of dramas that take the reader through Ronna Russell's rigid fundamentalist childhood, the disgrace of her preacher father, her sexual explorations, and the slow decline and dissolution of her marriage. Russell's sparing, matter-of-fact prose is the perfect vehicle for this autobiography, offering a counterpoint to the often painful and shocking events described. Her seamless chronological shifts from childhood to adulthood and back remind the reader of the ways in which the past informs the present and abuse of any kind is sticky and enduring. Though Russell's confessions ultimately celebrate the capacity of women to survive and thrive, they are never preachy, or self-indulgent. Indeed, the book opens with the most sizzling sex scenes I've ever read. This is a book to devour at one or two sittings, then pass on to your bestie!

-Dr. Claire Robson, Author of *Love in Good Time* and *Writing for Change*

The Uncomfortable Confessions of a Preacher's Kid is a brave, unflinching look at what happens when secrets go untold and questions go unasked. Ms. Russell's no-nonsense voice carries the reader into the dark crevices of TWO nuclear families living in hypocrisy and shame. And when she finally finds her own way into the light, she gets there in the most unconventional way. *Uncomfortable Confessions* is a must-read for all of us who have ignored what was right under our noses.

-Cami Ostman, Editor of *Beyond Belief: The Secret Lives of Women in Extreme Religion* and author of *Second Wind: One Woman's Midlife Quest to Run Seven Marathons on Seven Continents*

Ronna writes with an honesty that is refreshing and authentic. Her conversational writing style draws you in and keeps you reading. Her story is at times painful, but her wittiness and raw humor shine through.

-Amber Garza author of *For the Win*

To Steve

xoxo

Contents

We're our own dragons as well as our own heroes,
And we have to rescue ourselves from ourselves.
-Tom Robbins *STILL LIFE WITH WOODPECKER*

Author's Note

I was raised the daughter of a preacher in the cult of the United Pentecostal Church, an oppressed and repressed environment that never felt right. The following stories are an exploration of different times of life, not necessarily told in chronological order, taking the reader back to early childhood and through events which set the stage for later decisions. The first chapter takes place as my marriage is falling apart and I have an affair that allows me to reclaim my sexual freedom.

The memories in these pages are my own. I cannot tell or interpret anyone else's story or experience, nor would it be fair for me to try. Others may remember occurrences differently or have had different reactions to them. All names have been changed, except when used by permission.

Acknowledgements

My deepest gratitude to everyone who has helped me along this journey and those who have put up with me while I traveled. To Cami Ostman, my insightful and patient writing coach who never let me get away with any bullshit, Rebecca Mabanglo-Mayor, Anneliese Kamola and all the writers of The Narrative Project whose feedback and friendship kept me moving forward. My editor, Susanna Barlow, who straightened things out ahead of schedule and under budget, and Dr. Ken Bangs and Reagan Rothe at Black Rose Writing for giving me a chance. Dear friends who read the pieces and told me not to quit-Amber Garza, Scot Lloyd, Rebecca Golling, Ariel Larson, Claire Robson; Malerie Plaugher, for your unending encouragement and curiosity; the ex-Christian community who remind me that my voice helps them on their own path, you know who you are. To my sisters, Karissa Hopkins and Susan Paynter, and my dearest Mama, Donna Fisher, you are beautiful inside and out. Thank you for letting me tell my story. Cody, Emily, Jenny and Henry, you are the pieces of my heart walking the earth. I could not be prouder of the people you have grown up to be or more grateful for the love you show me and each other.

And Steve, most of all.

The Uncomfortable Confessions of a Preacher's Kid

Part One

Chapter 1
Vlad

Vlad gave his profile serious consideration. He answered all the questions, shared personal preferences, and was forthright about what he sought. He had posted one tasteful photo of himself sitting by a creek with his muscular back and shoulders framed against the rushing water. A hint of gray hair curled at the nape of his neck, his face obscured. Mercifully and to his credit, no dick pics were posted. Vlad sent a message my first day on the website, and we began to chat. His dry wit, obvious intelligence, and a desire to meet me all worked in his favor. Personal email addresses were exchanged soon after.

Vlad was seeking a married cohort to keep a secret with; someone with as much to lose as he did. He felt there was some degree of safety in that arrangement. Vlad's communication was spotty at first. He was slow to respond at times and explained the lengths he went to, to not get caught by his wife, which included using a separate SIM card for his phone. They both had successful businesses and he seemed to be an attentive husband and father. But when no one was looking, he switched out his SIM card and solicited sex with strangers online. Every time I logged onto the website, he showed up as "Active."

I was shocked to realize that married men did this kind of thing, that their need for sex led to behavior this calculating. It was news to me that phones could have more than one SIM card. I had permission to play, an arrangement worked out with my ever-more-distant husband, which allowed me to feel an edge of moral superiority, but I felt guilty that I was participating in Vlad's deception. Not guilty enough to stop, however. I decided his marriage was not my responsibility. I wasn't cheating, he was. Or so I told myself.

Vlad was cocky, funny, and sarcastic; attractive and arrogant. He vowed to have me begging for cock (I have the pussy, you beg, I said. He did not back down.). I issued a list of requirements which he promptly agreed to, condoms and I can't remember what else. We had a date almost planned when I put him off. I got nervous. How do affairs work, even when not having to sneak? There were a lot of details to consider: when and where and who pays for what. I did not have money for hotel rooms, and it was not a date. Vlad lived a couple of hours away, so some planning was required. This was not going to be a quick hook-up. How would I explain my absence? Could I do this?

Also, I was just plain chicken and not sure about Vlad, anyway. I thought he might piss me off in person because he was such a know it all. Sensing my hesitation, he lulled me with romantic memories of past lovers. We talked, via email, about what turns us on. He loved my descriptions of the way doggie style makes me feel fucked, full, taken. I admitted to liking the idea of being spanked; he did not forget that. He teased but was never mean, and cracked jokes constantly. We exchanged impromptu, Dr. Suess-style dirty poetry.

I would fuck you in a bar
I would fuck you in a car
I would fuck you here or there
I would fuck you anywhere...

Delightfully silly, but pretty bad as poetry goes. I was relieved to have someone to laugh with, an escape from the clenched jaw tension between myself and my husband. I was charmed by Vlad's attention, as I sat in my office with the door closed, ignoring my family.

We set a date to meet at a hotel in White Rock, just over the US/Canada border. Vlad was very picky about hotels; they must have good reviews. He wouldn't want something cheesy. He picked one out, a place across from the ocean with decent reviews, and reasonable rates, which he, fortunately, agreed to pay. I arrived first and sat on the couch in the lobby by the fireplace, waiting. Antsy. Fidgeting with the handle of my green leather bag, stocked with lingerie, condoms, lube, and my vibrator. I was not making any assumptions about Vlad being able to bring me to orgasm. Most men did not seem to know where to start, and I did not know what to tell them, not that anyone had ever asked.

Vlad texted, "I'm here. Meet me in the diner."

I walked out of the hotel lobby into the balmy, seaside air, and sunshine and into the tiny, clustered L-shaped diner next door, packed with people and reeking of fried onions. I nervously scanned the customers. Vlad was not among them. As I turned to leave, there he was on the sidewalk, squinting into the sun looking lost, searching for the diner's entrance. I stepped out through the grimy glass door and called his real name. He stopped, turned, and flashed his thousand watt smile. Vlad's electric blue eyes lit up as he walked toward me.

"Nice to meet you," he said, reaching out to shake my hand.

I laughed, sidestepped his hand, and put my arms around his waist, pulling him in for a hug.

"Hi," I smiled, discarding my nervousness with touch.

He kissed me, all tongue. He was already hard and kept kissing me, right out on the sidewalk, right there in front of the diner windows. Sweet. Delicious. I stopped trying to kiss back and let him lick the inside of my mouth, amused at his excitement. I wondered if the diners were watching.

"Let's go," I laughed when he took a breath.

We walked back into the labyrinthine hotel hallways, through the ice room, around the corner, kissing in the elevator, knees wobbling, around another corner, fumbling with the key. Excitement, nervousness, and panic all vied for space in my chest. I refused to think about what I was doing. Once inside, we found a lush, beautiful room with a luxurious bed; not cheesy at all.

And then, God almighty. I stripped that man of his clothes to discover a physique made entirely of muscle with a long tongue and a long cock stuck on in the right places. Just muscle, cock, and tongue. I knew he was an elite biker and skier but hadn't thought about what that meant. It meant zero body fat. Jesus. He rippled.

We sat on the bed, total strangers, face-to-face for the first time, and completely naked. He brought condoms as requested, and was willing to use them, although neither of us wanted to.

I said, "I don't know how hard you play."

He insinuated, vaguely, that this was his first actual encounter in fourteen years of marriage. He had been vasectomized long ago. Condoms did not seem necessary. He obviously wasn't worried about it, so I figured we be would okay. I did not present any danger to him.

Vlad was lying, of course. He played hard, and I took an awful chance, not using protection. I came to realize over the next couple of months that Vlad had a high degree of success online. He could get women into bed anywhere, anytime, and had a long history of unfaithfulness. He had probably never been faithful to his wife. During one of our many conversations, he described biking through a park and seething with desire as he watched young women stretched out on towels in the grass. I wondered at that pent-up desire. How many men feel that away, desperate to fuck? I felt that way. Did other women?

We turned our attention to each other. I began with long, slow, get-to-know-you licks. Vlad's cock announced itself, long and hard, big red knob angled away from his belly at the head.

He murmured, "This isn't fair," and pulled me around in one smooth motion.

His first lick, from ass to clit was electric. I gasped at the current that woke my body. I hadn't been touched like this, ever. We set about to exploring, heat building quickly. By the time he entered me, I could only moan.

"You are so responsive," he murmured.

"*Well, Jesus H. Christ, that tongue, those hands, that cock all seemingly made of fireworks or something, after twenty years of neglect,*" I thought, unable to formulate words.

"Uuuhhhhh," I said.

He rubbed my back as we faced the mirror on the closet door, holding each other's gaze in the reflection, eyes sparkling with playfulness. Vlad raised his hand and swatted the hell out of my ass, still holding my gaze. Startling, fabulous sensation. I burst out laughing and turned to inspect the damage. We stared at his handprint, wondering if it would go away anytime soon or if I would have to change my clothes in secret for a week. Even with our open arrangement, I did not want to advertise my activities to my husband. This was for me.

I was on top, suddenly conscious of my stomach skin, hovering low over his body as if somehow I could hide that troublesome wattle, stretched out from babies, as it hung embarrassingly. Vlad's face cringed when his hand brushed against its looseness.

I had trouble finding a rhythm because of his thrusting and put a hand on his hip to stop his movements. He relaxed. I controlled the fuck and forgot about my stomach skin.

"I don't want to come yet," he whispered.

"Tell me when to stop," I breathed.

"Stop," he moaned, looking at me with glazed eyes.

"Do you want to get together again?" he asked, with a catch in his throat.

"Yes, do you?" I smiled.

"Yes," he answered.

Vlad grasped my hips and turned us over. He entered me doggie style.

"Is this what you meant by feeling fucked?" he asked, moving slowly.

I tried to say yes, but it came out in a whimper. Vlad came, long and slow.

When he finished, I lowered to my stomach, keeping him inside as he laid stomach-down on my back. Eventually, we extricated ourselves, had some cheese and crackers, and took a nap. He did not snore at all. When we woke up, he was hard again and fucked me from behind, on our sides, his head tucked under my arm as I twisted toward him. He sucked my nipple while I lay there, my left leg wrapped around his, amused.

"Having fun back there?" I asked.

"Yes, just be my sex toy," Vlad grinned.

"Mmmm, ok," I sighed, relaxing into his body.

He fucked me from a ninety-degree angle, which started a vaginal orgasm rolling that would not quit. I used my vibrator while he sucked my toes; a revelation of sensuality. I had never comprehended that toe sucking could be sexy, instead of dumb and kind of gross. Not so. Whole toes in his hot, wet mouth while my orgasm built. I came with my vibrator while he kissed me, all tongue and wet, devouring kisses. Shreds of my sanity were left after that. While I came again with the vibe, he gave up waiting for me to ever be done and got in the shower.

That was the first time in my entire life I had ever spent the afternoon in bed with a man, been rolled around and loved from head to toe, with no thoughts of anything or anyone else, with nowhere else to be. The first time my forty-six-year-old body had ever received that much attention. Heaven.

Vlad put me back in my body and back in touch with my sexual self. All of my parts came alive. He was an expert in technique, and our chemistry was explosive. It is fair to say this was the best sex I had ever had to that point, by a lot. The first time I had ever felt ecstasy.

I also learned I could keep my emotional distance; that I could enjoy a sexual connection without emotional need. Expectations had always been front and center in my sexual relationships. That was the deal, reinforced with a heavy hand by the Pentecostal Church of my childhood. Body equals soul. Sex equals love. If I give my body, I am owed devotion. Technically, the church said emotions were supposed to come first-body sharing came afterward-and only within the bounds of marriage, but I had always done it backward, colliding like a wind-up toy into the wall of indifference from past lovers. And husband. After years of sexual disinterest from him, I needed to be fucked well, to feel heat and passion and desire; to have the flirting, the attention, and the laughter. But I did not need entanglements or drama. Since I was not planning to divorce and was not willing to break up my family, I did not want someone who expected anything from me outside of bed. I needed to feel desired, to feel worthy of desire, and then to feel the desire itself in the heat of his touch. Vlad's passion for me was like a mirror. This is what was missing, the connection between my body and another.

Sex with Vlad was not reciprocal; my skills were no match for his, and anytime I tried to take the initiative we faltered, so I laid back and let him lead. In bed with Vlad was the only place in my life I was not in charge. For a few hours at a time, he held off the increasing pressure that choked my days, as my marriage deteriorated.

He did get attached to me and brought up being together, an idea I shot down without hesitation. We were in another hotel room, a few weeks later. I had gotten there first, as usual. I suspect he stacked his dates up and went from one tryst to another because this time he brushed his teeth upon arrival and still tasted like pussy. He had to have a reason to be out for hours. After this romp, he had to go for a hike so that he could go home with muddy boots because that is what he told his wife was going to do. Vlad did not hike like an average person. He climbed straight up mountainsides without trails, using a machete to hack his way to the top. We were in bed, post-hot sex, lying side by side. Vlad complained about his wife; her intense drive, her lack of interest in sex, constant dissatisfaction, and nitpicking; her focus on appearances, vanity, and pettiness. On and on he whined.

"The very things about her that were attractive to you in the first place are the things driving you crazy now-her looks, ambition, and drive," I snapped, yanking the sheet over my breasts. When had I become his marriage counselor?

"Yeah..." he sighed in agreement and while staring at the ceiling, tentatively probed, "What about us?"

"*God, no.*" I thought. "We would drive each other nuts," I blurted out, surprised and somewhat horrified at the question.

"Yeah, that's true," he sighed again and did not meet my gaze.

I did not want Vlad out of bed. I sure as hell wasn't going to leave my husband and disrupt my family for him. I did not want him to love me. No more words were said as we drifted into a doze.

Later, as I sat in his lap eating strawberries, Vlad said, "You know, the thing that would bother my wife the most, if she found out about us, is who you are. 'HER?' she would say. Because, you're not *gorgeous*, you know."

He reached for a strawberry as he spoke, avoiding my gaze again. I froze in his lap.

Meaning I am not pretty at all, not attractive enough for his wife to understand or excuse the affair. He was cheating on her with someone plain. There could be no forgiveness for that. His words were retaliation for not wanting him, and they did sting. I did not respond, leaving his words to hang in the air. In truth, I did not give a shit what he thought about my face. His cruel words were empty. I already knew Vlad was an asshole.

Was I done with him now? I thought. *Almost.*

Soon after, Vlad wanted to spend the night together and went to great lengths to arrange to be away from home overnight. We discussed my desire to orgasm during intercourse without a vibrator, and I was pretty sure I knew how to make it happen. I would need a drink to relax. He showed up with the makings for screwdrivers, which I thought appropriate, and we got to it in the same White Rock hotel room where we first met.

When the cocktail had taken effect, I pushed Vlad up against the headboard, straddled him, and rode his cock to an explosive orgasm. I was fantastically vocal. He wondered in awe if the neighbors heard. If there were guests in the next room, they heard.

I hated sleeping next to him, uncomfortable with the intimacy of sharing the deepest hours of the night. We did not belong together. I had gotten what I needed from Vlad. We had sex a couple more times in the morning, and I drove away with a smile and a wave good-bye. Somehow we both knew it was over; we did not contact each other after that. I never saw him again; did not want to, did not need to.

Chapter 2
The Rapture and Other Bedtime Stories

All children are hostages of their parents; the complete dependence of babies and parental responsibility for their survival sets it up that way. Within the United Pentecostal Church, control is taken a few steps further. The Bible is considered the rulebook for parenting and is taken literally. Where biblical instructions are vague, interpretations are decided by the church for its members, who are expected to comply without question. UPC parents withhold exposure to the secular world from their children to create a closed circle of information, because exploration of any kind is a slippery slope to nonbelief. To do otherwise would be irresponsible. Nothing matters more than salvation; the punishment for sin is an eternity spent in Hell. No loving parent wants that for their child.

The second coming of Jesus Christ was a real and present danger. The Rapture was simultaneously presented as an event to anticipate, a great escape from life's trials and tribulations, and an existential threat. Jesus might return at any moment, with one deafening trumpet blast by way of announcement, to whisk the saved up to Heaven in the blink of an eye. The unsaved would be left on earth, which would become Hell, complete with Satan, fire, and demons. Those unfortunate souls left behind would burn forever without respite. Descriptive stories of Hell were meant to frighten the uncommitted into salvation and keep the already-saved on the straight and narrow. Those who had received the Holy Ghost could be excited about their impending escape from the life they shunned. Those without had better get saved right away or risk spending eternity in fiery doom. The Rapture was a common theme for Sunday night sermons. The Rapture was the reason for everything.

All humans were going to Hell when the Rapture took place, except for the handful of earth's population who belonged to the United Pentecostal Church, and had successfully completed the steps to salvation. No other Christians of any sort, not even other fundamentalists if they were not part of the UPC sect, were going to Heaven. Period. Not Baptists, nor Methodists, nor Lutherans, and especially not those pagan Catholics with their idolatry of Mary and the Saints.

"Mama," I contemplated in the car on the way home from church, "what about people in other countries who had never heard about Jesus. Are they going to Hell?" I knew the missionaries Daddy sent to faraway places could not get to everyone.

Mama explained over her shoulder, "Yes, it's too bad for those people. Their ancestors rejected God in the past, and so they never received the word of Jesus first-hand."

She was matter-of-fact about it, but her eyebrows were raised all the way up making cornrows on her forehead, so I knew she was serious.

I scooted back against the seat, stunned and sobered, as streetlights blurred by in the dark. This seemed unfair to me. Innocent people all around the world were going to burn in Hell forever and ever without having the chance to choose Jesus. Sinners who rejected him on purpose had it coming, such as our relatives who were backsliders, but to never have heard about him and still have to burn forever seemed cruel. I felt relieved and lucky to know the truth, and happy that Daddy made it possible for people all over the world, at least some of them, to hear about Jesus and be saved, too. I did not want any of those ignorant, brown-skinned foreigners in other countries to go to Hell. I worried that I was not saved, but I knew what to do.

The constant fear of the Rapture could only be assuaged by being saved in a specific way. Salvation was a three-step recipe: repentance, submersion baptism in Jesus' name, and speaking in tongues, in that order.

Step One: Repent for your sins by sincerely apologizing to God for every wrong thing you had ever done. This was easy and self-explanatory. Repentance could also be done on an ongoing, as-needed basis. God was forgiving, just ask.

Step Two: Baptism was more involved, as it required volunteering to be dunked by a qualified preacher, usually the pastor or a visiting evangelist. Baptisms performed in the name of the Father, Son, and Holy Ghost were invalid because this was an acknowledgment of the Trinity. According to the Oneness doctrine of the United Pentecostal Church, all three entities were one and the same. They were not three separate beings and to believe otherwise was blasphemy. The wording had to be correct, or the baptism did not count. People who had been baptized elsewhere under the Trinity had to be re-baptized in Jesus' name when they joined the UPC and got saved for real.

Step Three: Speaking in tongues was by far the most challenging requirement. Repentance and baptism were achieved easily enough of your own free will, but receiving the Holy Ghost, a gift bestowed by God to those deemed worthy, was beyond human control. Getting the Holy Ghost happened to salvation seekers during periods of free-form worship, such as altar calls toward the end of Sunday night services. Praying out loud with hands raised and eyes closed was the starting position. The Holy Ghost would take over the seeker's surrendered tongue, and temporarily speak through them in another language if their heart was right with God. I do not think the Holy Ghost would activate vocal cords during silent prayer. In retrospect, I'm not clear on that point. Worshippers did not begin to speak Italian or Vietnamese, of course. Speaking in tongues was gibberish; it is referred to in religious research as glossolalia, which I assume to be a psychological condition. Once the Holy Ghost had taken over the prayer's ability to speak, salvation was complete. Any sins committed in the future could be rectified with repeated repentance. Repetition of all three steps was not necessary, although regular, or at least occasional, speaking in tongues was expected. Routine maintenance by constant vigilance of behavior, attitude, and appearance, as well as regular church attendance, and tithing ten percent of your income, was all that was required to remain saved.

I was a rule follower and saw no reason to put off salvation. Going to Hell was not a risk I was willing to take. I repented for my kindergarten sins by chanting, "I repent for my sins in Jesus' name" several times, leaning over the altar with my eyes closed and my face buried in my hands. My palms were hot and sweaty, and I could smell my trapped breath. I wasn't sure what my sins were, exactly, but I sure was sorry. The Bible said we were all born with sin, so at least I had to repent for the sins I came with. Afterward, I told Daddy I wanted to be baptized because that was the next step. He smiled when I asked, his handsome face alive with delight. When Daddy was happy with me, my heart nearly burst. His lap was the center of the universe, his approval like the sun. I adored him.

Daddy baptized me. Most people had to be baptized by the pastor, but because Daddy was a preacher, too, he was qualified to ask God to wash my sins away. When Sunday evening church service was over, Daddy, Mama, and I snuck up the back stairs to the baptismal, which was situated above and behind the pulpit for full dramatic effect. Baptisms were usually a public production, but Daddy kept the red, velvet curtains closed. No one knew we were in there. Mama helped me change into a long, white robe in the dressing room with only my underwear on underneath and led me into the baptismal chamber where Daddy was waiting.

"Are you ready?" he asked with a tender, excited smile on his face. His hazel eyes shone with happiness behind silver frames. He had taken off his suit jacket and rolled up the sleeves of his crisp, white shirt.

I nodded and took his outstretched hand with complete trust. His hand felt warm and steady. He held onto me as I walked down the white steps. I knew he wouldn't let me slip. As I descended, tepid water soaked into my robe and the fabric clung to my legs. Daddy stood by the side of the tank, one strong hand on the back of my head, and one on my forehead. He closed his eyes to pray.

"Father, we come to you tonight to dedicate Ronna's life to you, Lord. Thank you for your love, for dying on the cross for our sins. Thank you for her love for you. Thank you, Jesus," he intoned solemnly.

Daddy helped me hold my nose, clasping his right hand over mine, and dipped me straight back into the water. As the back of my head broke the surface, I heard him announce, "I baptize you in the name of Jesus!" and the water closed over my face. He pulled me up again right away, laughing with joy. I smiled up at him, happily meeting his gaze.

Later, in the side aisle of the auditorium, he showed me off to another adult, my damp, towel-dried hair hanging heavy and snarled down my back. Daddy was proud of me. Soon I would be ready to go to Heaven, too. I wanted to be there with him.

Now, to get the Holy Ghost. No one could help me with that, not even Daddy. I prayed and prayed and prayed every single Sunday night. One time, it seemed like I got very close to speaking in tongues. I had been at the altar on my knees for a long time in the small auditorium after children's church. My skirt was tucked up around my legs to keep my knees covered as I listed sideways onto my hip, tired arms propped on the bench. Adults surrounded me, suit jackets and dresses whispering as they moved, their soft, gentle, encouraging prayers in my ears.

"Let go, let Jesus have your tongue, turn it over to Jesus," they chanted while touching my back and holding up my slumping arms. "That's riiight, that's riiight."

"Aww, honey. Oh, she's just right there," they said to each other over my head. "Come on, darlin'."

Dry sobs shook my body as I waved my arms weakly in the air. "Jesus, Jesus, Jesus..." I begged.

I stammered, trying to find the right balance between speaking aloud and keeping my tongue loose for Holy Ghost control, if only it would take over. I felt desperate and confused, wondering what I was doing wrong. I had followed the steps. I did not ever sin on purpose. I even crossed that one swear word out of my diary and dated it so Jesus would know I meant it. I could not go to Heaven until the Holy Ghost took over my tongue. Why wouldn't Jesus save me? I was trying so hard.

One of the adults gave a sympathetic laugh and said, "Poor lil' thing." I felt their hands leave me and the prayers stop. Their warm presence evaporated as they wandered away. They had given up on me for the night. I opened my eyes, squinting in the sudden light. The auditorium was too bright, and my legs were numb.

I could not figure out what else to do. All the other church kids had the Holy Ghost already. I should be a good candidate for salvation since everyone else in my family was saved and ready to go. Why would Jesus save my sisters and not me? I was embarrassed, a misfit sinner, and did not know why.

Being unsaved was terrifying all the time. Our family visited Brother and Sister Thorp's house. Brother Thorp was a big, loud preacher with a booming laugh and Sister Thorp was tiny and watchful. Sister Thorp and Daddy taught Bible studies together and were close friends, both short, good-looking, and smart. I stood in the Thorp's driveway at the open trunk of our car, reaching in to grab my bag. My back was to the street, which made me nervous. I never liked to have any open space behind me, always preferring to have my back to the wall. A car horn blasted right behind me. I jumped in fright, dropped my bag, and whirled around, eyes wide and heart pounding. Brother Thorp hopped out of his car howling with laughter.

"You thought it was the trumpet of Jesus and you are not ready!" he whooped and strode into the house, cackling all the way. I stood beside the car, humiliated by my lack of salvation until my heart rate returned to normal. I did not get the joke and was ashamed that he saw through my fear. *How could he tell I was not saved just by looking?*

When I was nine years old and my sisters, Susan and Karissa, were teenagers, Daddy decided he needed to be home more. He had worked for UPC Headquarters Foreign Missions Department for a long time and was tired of traveling. Daddy told Mama she had been a good mother to us in our early childhood, but it was time for him to take over raising the kids. He would be home all the time now and did not need her help. From then on, she would need to check with him first before making any decisions regarding my sisters and me. Mama was surprised to be relieved of her parental duties but acquiesced to his wishes without dissent. The Bible, the indisputable word of God, ordered her to be submissive to him. That meant all the time. Mama told me decades later that she knew she had abdicated her role as our parent by accommodating Daddy's demand for control, but at the time she let it happen, to keep the peace. Standing up to him would be the start of World War III, as she put it.

Daddy accepted a job as vice-president of Jackson College of Ministries, a small Bible school owned and operated by the First Pentecostal Church in Jackson, Mississippi. Mama did not want to live in Mississippi, but went along with the plan, because Daddy said God called him to do it. When God gave Daddy a calling Mama had to trust him because God spoke directly to men first. Susan and Karissa were upset to leave their friends in St. Louis. My bouncy excitement annoyed them; moving seemed like an adventure to me. What did I know?

Due to real estate market luck, we moved into a stately neighborhood built in an old pecan orchard, where every house had a one-acre yard, aptly named Pecan Acres. Perfectly manicured lawn hugged the curve of the sweeping driveway all the way down to the broad, tree-lined street. Our yard was so big Daddy had to buy a riding lawnmower, to his delight. Dreamy moonlight shone through the fluttering, silvery leaves of the pecan trees at bedtime. I had never seen anything like it.

We arrived in the Deep South on a pedestal. Daddy's installation as vice-president of Jackson College of Ministries was a big deal. His job was to whip the floundering school into shape. Expectations were high. Daddy led our family into the soaring, white auditorium on our first Sunday night service at the First Pentecostal Church. I gazed at the triple sectioned expanse of padded, pea green pews spanning the immense sanctuary, separated by broad aisles of matching green carpet. My eyes rose to the balcony. Every seat was filled. This church was a lot bigger than the one in St. Louis.

We all followed Daddy in single file to a pew five rows back on the left, and I perched on the high, cushioned seat, safely ensconced between Mama on my left, and Karissa and Susan on my right. Mama smoothed her skirt, tucking the hem behind her knees, panty-hosed legs crossed at the ankle. She folded her hands in her lap and rubbed the empty ring finger of her left hand. Not even wedding rings were allowed in Jackson. Daddy sat by the aisle. Coarse upholstery scraped the backs of my thighs through my tights, pulling them down with even more veracity than the wooden pews had at the old church. I would never win the battle between tights and pews.

My feet swung in new, black patent leather Mary Janes, not quite reaching the floor. From my seat, I could see a tall, wooden pulpit with a built-in microphone, flanked by music pits filled with instruments and musicians: piano, organ, electric organ, drums, harp, guitars, electric guitars, and bass. A row of throne-like chairs sat behind the pulpit for extra preachers. A tiered choir loft rose behind the thrones stretching all the way up to the curtained baptismal. Up further still, two small balconies overlooked the platform from either side, where young men confidently handled trumpets and saxophones. I scanned their faces to see if any of them were cute.

After opening hymns, Brother Weston, the pastor, and the president of JCM announced, "Here with us tonight is Brother Donald Fisher and his beautiful family. Come on up, all-a-y'all, and join me on the platform."

He turned, opening his arms in our direction, welcoming us to the stage with a huge smile. The congregation applauded.

Daddy led the way as we stood and filed out from between the pews. I followed Mama's familiar, polyester rear up the green, carpeted platform steps to the left of the pulpit, our family lined up in front of 1500 people spread across the vast auditorium, as if for inspection. Brother Weston introduced us one by one, choosing me last.

"What's your name, darlin'?" he asked, as he held the microphone down to my mouth,

"Ronna," I spoke into the mic.

"How old are ya, Ronna?" he continued in a friendly voice.

"Niiiine," I drawled.

"She has a Southern accent already!" Brother Weston punted to the crowd, who laughed in response.

The Fishers had arrived. I was surprised to be on display. Now all of these people knew my name, but I did not know anyone. I was surprised to be a sudden celebrity and had no idea what that might mean. Daddy was even more important here than he was in St. Louis. He had a big job to do, and Mama was going to help him. Susan, Karissa, and I were there to be examples. Of what I never knew.

Karissa and I adopted Southern accents upon arrival in Jackson. The twang was not difficult to mimic and saved an enormous amount of hassle and teasing for sounding like Northerners. Anyone not from the Deep South was considered a Northerner and could never fit in. Speaking with a Southern drawl was a quick way to fend off ridicule. Our adaptation drove Mama and Daddy crazy because, they said, the slow slur sounded stupid. Susan thought Southern accents were ridiculous and did not bother. She regularly came home from high school, howling with laughter that "on" and "own" and "aunt" and "ain't" were considered homonyms, among other linguistic transgressions. I heard teenagers at church refer to black people as niggers. I had never heard the term used before but knew it was derogatory. Racism has an undeniable ring. While I was eager to adopt the language of my new home, I did not understand its history. Everyone I encountered was white, even though I lived in a city whose population was largely mixed. No people of color lived in our neighborhood or went to my school or church. I heard nothing of the Civil Rights movement or Martin Luther King, Jr.; knew nothing about the Confederate flags on display. I did not know active members of the Ku Klux Klan attended the same church I did.

A few weeks after settling into our new home, I walked to the end of our driveway, got on the school bus, and was delivered to fourth grade in a segregated school, much like the one I left behind. I hadn't realized how at home I felt before, going to the same elementary school Susan and Karissa attended. Kids in St. Louis were used to me. I was a good girl and a good student, which had always been enough to get along, even though I dressed weird.

Socializing at school was not allowed. All other kids were from sinner families and must be kept at arms' length. They were not okay to befriend, as they would be a bad influence with their televisions and blue jeans, and goodness knows what other perversions. I was, however, allowed to witness to them or invite them to church, so that they could be saved.

A girl named Laura sat with me at lunch.

"Want to come to church with me?' I asked.

"Sure, I'll ask my Dad," Laura chirped. In Mississippi, everyone went to church somewhere.

Next day:

Laura: I can't go because my dad said your church is weird.

Me: You can tell your dad that I am not weird.

Next day:

Laura: I told my dad what you said. I'm grounded.

She stopped sitting by me at lunch.

Girls huddled on the playground, discussing their preference of Cassidy Brothers. I hung back at the edge of the circle, silent and shy, with no idea who the brothers were. Sarah, with freckles and glasses, turned to me, "Which one do you like?"

I peeked over a classmate's shoulder at her open magazine showing two handsome faces, fortunately, labeled. *Sean obviously*, I thought, but shrugged and did not respond because I was too embarrassed for words to come out of my mouth.

Being at school felt as though I had been painted red and told not to stand out. School happened around me. Academics were easy enough, and good grades were expected at home, but every child understands the real work of school is social. Sometimes the two overlapped, creating an insurmountable level of confusion. Any acknowledgment offered to me was refused on my behalf. My fifth-grade teacher chose me to be the hall monitor, an honor given to responsible kids. Mama wrote the teacher a note declining the opportunity because I was too bossy already and this responsibility would give me a venue I did not need. My personality was not good enough. To be fair, she probably did me a favor. The hall monitor was always resented. When the teacher told the girls in class (me) to leave our little dresses at home and wear blue jeans the next day for field day, Mama wrote another letter explaining that because of our religious beliefs that wasn't going to happen. I saw the teacher's frustration, the set of her mouth, as she tossed Mama's letter aside. I had seen that look before.

When the music teacher asked the class who had seen *Star Wars*, everyone raised their hands. Hmmm... I had seen stars outside at night... but that wasn't what she meant... I raised my hand along with everyone else and prayed for no follow-up questions. I began to keep my nose in a book as much as possible. Reading seemed like the safest option for getting through the day.

Socializing was more comfortable at church. At least I knew what everyone was talking about. On Sunday mornings, kids were divided by age for Sunday school classes. I sat with my designated group, at a table with the cool kids from the prominent church families, who allowed me to be peripheral for a while. For reasons I never understood, I became an outcast there, as well. These kids were multigenerational Mississippians, which was its own kind of club, and I was never going to be one them. They spent weekends in the backwoods with their extended families hunting, boating, four wheeling, and barbequing. Mississippi was their home. I remember the low, mocking voice behind my back at the Sunday school table that told me my time as part of the group was over. I ran the test of not sitting with the cool kids the next week to see if anyone noticed. They did not. Church kids had a lot of freedom, and the general vibe was pretty sexed-up, with heaping sides of backbiting and gossip. Dating started before puberty. Marriages between teenagers were not uncommon, especially if they had been caught having sex. I was in over my head with that crowd, anyway.

Daddy and Mama were uncomfortable with the cultural differences in Jackson and never interacted with church people. Daddy told Mama to never tell anyone in Jackson anything because they would talk about you behind your back as soon as you left the room. Social ostracism deepened as Mama and Daddy's discomfort and need for control grew. Their philosophy on childhood friendships was unusually strict, even by church standards. Free time before and after service was to be spent on my knees in the prayer room, not standing in the hall talking in clusters with other kids. Sitting by boys during church was forbidden, speaking to them at all prompted accusations of misbehavior from Daddy. I was not allowed to attend the church girl sleepovers, not old enough at ten or eleven when the invitations stopped coming. Asking to spend time with other girls was risky, especially if it was a spontaneous plan cooked up at church. Such a request might be met with rage, I never knew.

After children's church one summer Sunday night, Amy invited me to sleep over. I was excited, eager to ask permission. I saw Daddy outside the double doors of the fellowship hall and ran up to him. Amy and her father followed me.

"Daddy, Daddy, can I spend the night at Amy's house? Please?" I asked hopefully.

"What? No, I need you to come home tonight. You have to work in the office at the Bible school in the morning," he scowled, his jaw rippled dangerously.

I whirled back to Amy. "Oh, um, I'm sorry, I can't," I stammered. "I have to go home."

Daddy did not acknowledge Amy or her father, but grabbed me by the neck and steered me toward the exit, furious. I struggled to keep up with him, as his thick fingers dug into my skin, tightening on my neck. He hissed in my ear, "Don't you ever put me in that position again."

I had stepped out of line. I tried to turn to wave goodbye to Amy. She and her father stood staring at us with jaws dropped, as we barreled toward the door, Daddy's hand still gripping my neck like a vise. Somehow, I knew his reaction was not normal and was embarrassed that they witnessed it.

I was still trying to get the Holy Ghost every Sunday night, but I never went down to the altar at the front of the main auditorium. Going to the big altar in front of the entire congregation would have been a public admission of my failure to attain salvation and would risk the invasive and humiliating laying on of hands. The altar was for real sinners, not for people like me who hadn't gotten the Holy Ghost but were faithfully trying. I stayed between the pews during the altar call, even though sometimes the whining organ music seemed to be calling my name.

One Sunday night, a few years after moving to Jackson, the music was thumping, and the already-saved believers were dancing in the spirit. Sometimes, when the band and choir played pump-up music, the congregation remained calm and quiet until the oompa-oompa beat awkwardly petered out. This was disappointing, and I felt embarrassed for the choir. Other nights, like this one, the Holy Spirit moved, and the dependable shouters began to whirl around in the aisles, chests thrusting back and forth to the music, or shaking wildly from head to toe. Then the choir director would ramp it up, as he bounced on his elevated stand, increasing the volume and tempo to a frenzy with his hand signals.

Musical performances at the First Pentecostal Church in Jackson, Mississippi were no joke. There was a vast choir with outstanding vocalists and a chorale of the best singers. Soloists belted lyrics into spit-covered microphones while banging tambourines, all accompanied by an orchestra played by expert musicians. The choir director was a Grammy winner. That house rocked. When the gospel music swelled, and the beat thumped, the mood of the congregation moved to ecstasy, and it was impossible to remain still. Most people remained standing in the pews, clapping, singing, and swaying, watching the brave shouters who gave their bodies and hairdos over to the music.

This particular Sunday night, I felt brave in my new black and red dress with its fringed shawl, even though I did not have breasts to fill out the neckline. No one was paying attention to me as I begged again for the Holy Ghost and, since everyone else was doing it, I thought maybe shouting would help. The congregation was already in disarray, their humping bodies writhing in the aisles. *I'm not sure how to start,* I thought. *Do I dare?* I squeezed my eyes closed. I felt out the pew back in front of me against my stomach and the edge of my seat against the backs of my knees, for boundaries. I raised my hands in the air and began hopping lightly side to side, waving my arms around, and praying softly. *Here goes,* I thought, committed to the effort.

"Jesus, Jesus, I love you, Jesus," I chanted as I bounced around.

After a few moments of amateur shouting and keeping my mouth loose and open, no superpower infiltrated my body or tongue. I did not feel even a glimmer of Holy Spirit or anything other than my own awkward limbs and my shawl creeping up around my neck. I slowed my movements to a stop but kept my eyes closed, and arms raised, continuing to pray, so my efforts did not look fake. Gradually easing out of the stance, I lowered my arms, squinched my eyes open, and looked around. No one had noticed, except Mama. She was waiting for me to finish and sidled up to me, wrapping an arm around my shoulders.

"You don't have to shout to worship, Ronna. Only do it if it's real," she disapproved into my ear.

Mama did not like demonstrative shouting and was not comfortable with my participation. Shouting was for other people.

A traveling evangelist, Brother Spoke, had preached his signature sermon that night, full of terrifying tales of untimely deaths and tragic accidents of the unsaved. He always got the congregation worked up. Brother Spoke told stories of sinners who left the church without seeking salvation and then got hit by trucks or suffered some other gruesome demise, guaranteeing an eternity in Hell. He waxed eloquent about the torture and flames of Hell, and how those things would feel. I watched him tower over the podium, leaning into the microphone, his pompadour hair slicked back from his forehead, and his hooded eyes glowering with doom.

"I don't think we are going to see 1977," he forewarned.

It was 1976. That night in bed, I sang myself to sleep to shut out his voice, watching the full moon shimmer through the silver leaves of the pecan trees outside my window. I still wasn't saved. Time was running out. I wondered if the fire would be everywhere.

I had difficulty going to sleep most nights, but always on Sundays. Some preachers said the Rapture would save us all in the nick of time from the horrors prophesied in the Book of Revelations, that we would be saved from the never-ending lick of hot flames on flesh, from the apocalypse, when accused Christians would be drawn and quartered by four horsemen. Daddy explained that each horseman would hold onto one of our arms and legs and ride off in opposite directions until our bodies were ripped apart. I did not want to die that way. Daddy said he did not believe we were going to get out without a scratch; meaning he believed some of us would be tortured and killed for our beliefs before the Rapture rescued us, so he was no help getting to sleep. I wished he would be reassuring like the other preachers, but deep down I was afraid he was right. He was always right about everything. Those other preachers were trying to make everyone feel better, but torture was coming for us. Daddy said so.

The next Saturday morning, I slept in later than usual and awoke to silence. The house felt eerily empty as I stepped out of my bedroom. No one was there. The Rapture had taken place, and I was alone in Hell. This was always how Hell started in stories when sinners had the horrifying realization that they had been left behind. I ran down the hall, heart pounding, a silent scream bursting my throat. As I passed Karissa's open bedroom door, I saw her asleep under the covers. I stopped running, digging my toes into the carpet. I did not say a word, did not make a sound, as I stood in her doorway and watched her sleep. I held my breath, as my heart pounded in my ears. She had the Holy Ghost, and she was still here. Jesus had not come. I was not in Hell. Gradually, my heart rate slowed, the tightened scream in my throat melted away, and I went in search of breakfast, still shaking.

Another Sunday night, during post-sermon worship, I stood between the pews with my eyes closed and my arms raised, as always, waiting for the force.

"Love you Jesus Jesus love you Jesus" I chanted without enthusiasm. I was tired of trying. Tired of being scared.

The sounds of other worshippers, the come-to-Jesus organ music, and crooning singers sounded far away. No one stood near or laid hands on me; a solitary moment. I let the babble out, mimicking sounds I heard other people make when they spoke in tongues.

"Oh, shondalakalila ooo-shukimakilalala, hondalee, hondalee," I stammered.

As I forced gibberish out of my mouth, the deep, unsettling fear of being an unsaved faker hung like smoke from the fires of Hell. I opened my eyes, lowered my arms, and swallowed dryly. Peeked around. No one was watching me, not even Mama.

During the car ride home, I skootched up in the back seat so Mama and Daddy could hear me in front.

"I got the Holy Ghost tonight," I announced between their heads.

They seemed vaguely surprised and, perhaps, a little bit disbelieving.

"Really? You did?" Mama asked.

"Oh, well, that's great, Ronna," Daddy said with a little laugh and turned back to Mama to resume their conversation.

I guess they hadn't been as worried about it as I was. I settled back into my seat, unsure if my parents believed me, but relieved by their inattention to the matter. After the initial clutch of fear passed, I did not worry about my lie much. As a matter of fact, a load of pressure was off my mind because people soon stopped asking if I had gotten the Holy Ghost. I said yes when they did ask, and that was that. Word got around. I had been waiting for a real experience, but as it turned out, I only had to pretend.

Chapter 3
Loose Demons

As far back as I can remember, long before I faked my own salvation, I was always a thousand miles away inside my head. During sermons that seemed endless, I tilted my head back against the hard, varnished pew and stared up at the arched ceiling, training my eyes to follow the boards, searching for one without a seam-a beam made of a solid piece, as the preacher's voice droned. This preacher was preaching for a long time.

"Mama," I whispered, "Can I lay on the floor under the pew?"

"Ok, just this once," she whispered back.

I slipped onto the floor and lay down on my stomach. I could see rows and rows of shoes. A couple of rows back there was a pair of high, white heels with pointy toes and a covered button on the strap, instead of a buckle. I was fascinated by this view of disembodied feet. I turned over and saw with shock that someone, lots of someones, had stuck gum underneath the pew. That had to be a sin. We weren't even supposed to chew gum in church. I got bored on the floor and crawled back up onto the pew in between Mama and Daddy to watch my own private optical illusion of the preacher's head growing smaller and farther away as he talked and talked. His tiny head and minuscule, waving hands floated up and away. I tried it on the teenage boy who played the drums, but his face came back into focus because he was cute. My gaze wandered over to the other side of the auditorium where the teenagers sat, trying to spot the other cute boys.

Daddy leaned forward, cleared his throat, and began cleaning his fingernails. He always had silver fingernail clippers with a little tiny chain attached in his pocket. He listened while concentrating on his fingernails, which were always clean. Sometimes he scribbled notes rapidly on a yellow legal pad with a black pen during sermons, or even on the back of his hand if he did not have any paper. I could not read his scrawling cursive, but I knew his thoughts must be brilliant by the way his chin went sideways while he wrote.

Organ music began to thrum when the preacher finally gave the altar call, an invitation for sinners to come to the front of the church and pray for salvation, and I knew service was almost over. The organist crooned into the microphone:

Come home, come home
Ye who are weary, come home
Softly and tenderly, Jesus is calling
Calling, O sinner, come home

A young man, a stranger, walked forward and knelt at the altar. Men, including Daddy, moved from the congregation toward the front and gathered around him. All the women remained in their seats.

"What's going on, Mama?" I whispered, straining to see around the heads blocking my view.

"He is possessed by a demon," she whispered without opening her eyes. She always did that, answered me with her eyes closed, if I interrupted while she was praying.

I did not know how Mama could tell the man had a demon, but I knew demons were evil beings that carried out Satan's commands and sometimes took over sinners' bodies. People who were not saved did not have any protection against demons. The man at the altar was obviously a sinner because his long hair curled over his collar, unlike Pentecostal men who were not allowed to let their hair touch the tops of their ears. Every man in the congregation surrounded him, looking terribly concerned. They were determined to cast out the demon with the laying on of hands. Praying for God to cast out demons was always called the laying on of hands.

The preacher placed his entire hand on top of the sinner's forehead and prayed into his face, breath and spittle flying. The sinner's head wobbled back and forth under the preacher's palm. Then the preacher shoved his hand into the sinner's forehead with a sudden, single jab, as if to push the demon right out the back of his head by surprise.

"I rebuke you, in Jesus' name," he screamed.

There was not enough room on this guy's head for all the hands, so some of the men put their hands on his shoulders and back; the others paced in a circle, as he hunched over, face to the altar now. All the men closed their eyes and began to beseech God.

"Satan, I demand you flee this child of God, in the name of Jesus!"

"Demon, get thee out!"

"Release him by thebloodoftheLamb!"

"JesusJesusJesusJesus"

The men's prayers got louder and more intense, their hands shaking the man and pushing him down. Women watched and waited in the pews, praying urgently with hands raised. I hardly dared to breathe. *What is going to happen when the demon comes out?* I wondered to myself. *I bet it's gonna come out any second now. How could it hold onto that sinner's insides with all those prayers attacking it?*

The demon was going to be loose in the church. THEN WHAT? Where do loose demons go? What would it look like? Would it seek another sinner or try to escape? Was it going to climb inside ME or head straight for the door? I did not have the Holy Ghost, so I knew I was not protected. I imagined a dark shadow with eyes slithering across the carpet like smoke. Why were we all sitting here? The demon was going to COME OUT! Hightailing it for the door seemed reasonable, except it might intercept me on the way out. How fast do demons move when they are in a hurry? Maybe it would choose someone else if I sat very still.

I sat frozen in my pew, legs firmly tucked beneath my bottom, eyes wide. The prayers subsided into moans, back clapping, and shoulder hugs. The congregation began to filter out of the auditorium. I followed Mama to the vestibule where she chatted with Sister Rudd, while Brother Rudd slipped me a butterscotch candy from his pocket with a wink as he always did. No one said anything about the demon, so I guess it was gone. I did not see the sinner around anywhere.

Sister Green waddled up to me with a big toothy cackle, "Hahaha, when you were a baby you were so fat we called you Cadillac, the biggest body by Fisher! Hahahaha!"

"Oh, my word," Mama joined in. "The doctor made me put her on skim milk when she was twelve months old! She weighed twenty-two pounds!" Mama exclaimed, laughing and shaking her head as if she couldn't believe how fat I was.

I sucked my butterscotch but did not laugh because I had a little hot spot of embarrassment lodged in my throat. I hated being reminded I was a fat baby. I found Daddy and held his hand until it was time to go.

The next morning at the breakfast table, Susan asked, "Do you remember walking in your sleep last night?"

"What? No," I answered, puzzled.

"Daddy found you standing at the top of the basement stairs with your eyes WIDE OPEN, but you were SOUND ASLEEP," she announced. "Your eyes were all glassy, but you weren't really looking at anything. It was super weird! HA, HA! You don't remember? Daddy took you back to bed. You could have fallen down the stairs!"

I shook my head. I had no recollection of my middle of the night wandering. A titch of fear tripped my stomach as I realized I could not control what my body did while it slept. *What was wrong with me? Did the demon get inside?*

"You did that once before. Mama and Daddy found you in the corner of your room trying to climb up the wall. It was really weird," Susan commented with a snort, as she set her cereal bowl in the sink.

After breakfast, I climbed down the steep, wooden stairs to the basement, with a tight grip on the cold, metal rail. The musty, damp smell of underground filled my nostrils as I descended step by step. My favorite places were down there, Susan and Karissa's adjoining bedrooms and a red and white kitchen playhouse made for us by our grandad. I poked my head into Karissa's room. She had the best bedroom, with giraffe decals on the wall behind bamboo poles, and a pink and white butterfly bedspread with a canopy. She was still in bed.

"Can I sleep with you in your room tonight, Karissa? Pleeeeeeaaase," I begged, rubbing my fingers on her silky, pink comforter.

"You ask me that every day," she groaned from her pillow, the pungent smell of her greasy hair wafting up.

"Pleeeeeeaaase, pleasepleaseplease," I groveled.

"NononononoYESnonono," she smirked.

"You said yes! YOU SAID YES," I crowed and hopped around.

"I said no," she answered with finality.

"You guys, be quiet," Susan ordered, as she flipped back the love beads separating their bedrooms and marched over to the desk on Karissa's side. She popped the cassette deck open and flipped her tape over with a sharp clack. She was listening to Andrae Crouch and the Disciples again.

"Get up, Karissa, it's almost time to catch the bus," Susan whirled back into her room, as the strands of colored beads shimmied into place.

School marked the days until time to go back to church. The United Pentecostal Church did not fool around when it came to outlining the rules. Daily life was defined by the forbidden, the church's claws reached far beyond mandatory attendance of twice on Sundays and once on Wednesday night. Maintaining a sense of separateness from the world was easily accomplished as our appearance announced our affiliation wherever we went. Strict decrees regarding entertainment and leisure activities also set us apart. Church members were not allowed to play or watch sports of any kind; card playing, television, and movies were absolutely forbidden, secular books and music severely limited. Association with non-church members, including neighbors and family, was discouraged. All of these parameters were designed to keep us saved and to ward off temptation and thus, Satan himself. You could hardly be possessed by a demon while immersed in biblical teachings, which is why Sunday services were the focal point of every week. Sunday school classes were held in the morning, but Sunday evening services were the main event. They were mostly boring, sometimes terrifying, with random bouts of excitement. Demonic possession was unusual, but you never knew what was going to happen.

Brother Chekov, a wiry, tightly wound little man with horn-rimmed glasses and black, slicked-back hair, was leading worship service. Excitement pulsed the auditorium. He became moved by the Holy Spirit and briskly paced the platform in his shiny, blue suit while swinging a white hanky in circles above his head. He worshipped in bellows with his eyes squeezed shut, as organ music pumped in the background. I watched from my spot on the rigid, bottom-numbing pew, tucked in next to Mama, squirming as my tights slid down, binding my thighs at the crotch, and inching my underwear down. I could barely see over the back of the pew in front of me, but if I positioned myself just right, glimpses of Brother Chekov appeared in between the heads of the adults seated there. My heart swelled with pride when I spotted Daddy sitting up on the platform with the other preachers, in one of the chairs that looked like a throne, with his legs crossed. I watched until I could no longer bear the feel of my sliding tights. I pushed the toes of my shiny, black Sunday night shoes into the hymnal box on the pew back and gripped handfuls of white lace tights, bracing myself while raising my rear off the seat to pull my tights back up, simultaneously stretching chin to chest to keep from yanking my knee length hair when I lowered back down. I had this maneuver down.

"Hallelujah! Thank you, Jesus! Halle**LUUU**jah! Halleluuuuuujahhhhhhh!" Brother Chekov hollered, his hanky became a whirling, white flash as his pace quickened. "Stand up! Stand up if you need healing tonight! Jesus is gonna heal you RIGHT NOW! RIGHT NOW! Praise his holy name! Halleluuuuuujahhhhhhh!"

Mama stood up, her flowered skirt rustling over layers of slip and pantyhose. She closed her eyes and raised her hands up to her slim shoulders, her mouth moving in silent prayer.

My heart pounded with worry. Mama was sick? Since when? I patted her immovable, girdled hip.

"Mama, Mama, what's wrong?" I whispered, watching her face.

Mama turned her head to me without opening her eyes, "I'm constipated," she mouthed, her eyelashes damp with tears.

Eyes widening with surprise, I turned my attention back to the pulpit. I did not know Jesus could fix bowel movements. BMs, we called them. I guess you could ask him anything.

Without warning, Brother Chekov leaped from the top step of the platform, landed on his feet, and shot like a cannon down the aisle, right past my pew. I whipped my head around to watch, spellbound, as he sprinted to the back of the auditorium. The organist pumped faster, bouncing up and down on the bench. Ushers jumped to open the double swinging doors to the vestibule. Brother Chekov ran straight through without slowing down, careened through the foyer, and burst back through the doors on the other side of the auditorium with a bang. The ushers couldn't get there in time; the doors swung wildly in Brother Chekov's wake. I craned my neck to see him race back up the far aisle to the steps on the other side of the platform. He returned to pacing and swinging his hanky, calling out to Jesus at the top of his lungs. His forehead was shiny with sweat, but he wasn't out of breath.

"Praise Jesus, praise Jesus! Woooooooooo," he shouted while he paced. He had sprinted around the entire auditorium with his eyes closed, but he never tripped.

The musicians picked up the tempo further, as the Holy Spirit spread to some of the women in the congregation who stood up, arms raised, and their eyes closed, swaying to the music. Mama sat back down beside me, still praying with her eyes closed, but not making a sound. Sister Johnson started the shouting. Her body convulsed, quick chest thrust out, then back, arms waving in rhythm, her bosoms keeping time while her blond beehive hung onto her scalp for dear life.

"Ayiyiyiyiyi," she yodeled.

Her first convulsion took hold; more followed in quick succession, back and forth, back and forth, faster and faster. The pink, knit fabric of her requisite knee-length skirt and long sleeves strained against her voluptuous body. She began speaking in tongues and weeping, twirling and dancing in circles, bumping into people and pews. This was not demonic possession; she was being moved by the Holy Spirit. Everyone understood. Sister Johnson would have gone home with bruises, but someone guided her out into the aisle. Other women joined her. Their hairdos loosened bit by bit, bobby pins flew, littering the carpet.

Shouting your hair down was considered to be a good thing, if somewhat amusing. Some people were shouters, and some were not. Mama never shouted, but always sat with her eyes closed and hands folded in her lap, weeping and praying. Her lips moved as tears dripped down her contorted face, but I never knew why she was sad. Daddy never shouted, either. Sometimes he closed his eyes and prayed, but he never cried. He watched from his big chair on the platform, while I watched from my pew until the shouting wound down and we all went home.

Women's hair was left uncut, not even trimming was allowed. Married women were required to wear their hair up. Some women, like Mama, crafted a demure bun, pinned and tucked into place over her ears, just like Ma did in my favorite Little House on the Prairie books. Others used the opportunity to create towering concoctions of poofs, swirls, loops, and braids.

Underneath lurked many mysterious items used for bun foundation and height, such as hairbrush leavings, which were saved up and packed into the feet of old pantyhose to create blobs called "rats." Household items from oatmeal cans to maxi pads were used for stuffing, along with much teasing and Aqua Net. Hairdos were a Pentecostal art form; one of the few permitted decorations of self. I always thought Mama could put in a little more effort to make it interesting.

I got a lot of attention for my hair, which hung to my knees by kindergarten. Every Saturday afternoon, Mama washed my hair in the kitchen sink.

"Time to wash your hair!' she called to me from the back door. I was headed for the swingset now that my chores were done, but hairwash came first. Afterward, I was allowed to have a half piece of chewing gum and would be free to play.

I turned back and followed Mama into the kitchen.

"Hop up,' she said, holding her arms down to me.

I reached up, and she hoisted me onto the counter. Shampoo and conditioner waited by the faucet; a bath towel was folded across the sink's edge. Mama ran the hot water, checking the temperature with her wrist.

"Ok, the water is ready. Lay down," Mama instructed in her no-nonsense voice.

I swung my feet up onto the counter and lay back with my neck on the towel, lowering my hair into the sink, which it practically filled. Mama shampooed and conditioned my hair with firm, but gentle hands. I kept my eyes squeezed shut while she used the sprayer to rinse.

She wrung out my hair several times with her hands and helped me sit up while unfolding the towel across my shoulders and placing my wet hair on top of it in one smooth motion. Then she folded it up, capturing the wet hair inside and hung the ends across my shoulders, creating a heavy neck wrap of damp hair and towel which I wore until my hair had stopped dripping and was dry enough to comb out.

I ran out to the yard, where Susan and Karissa were playing tetherball with the neighbor kids, who were not allowed in the house because they were not Pentecostal. Susan was beating everybody again. I skirted the older kids and climbed onto the swingset to watch until my hair dried and Mama called me back in.

Mama sprayed my hair with detangler and began inching the snarls out as I braced myself against the pull of her big, green comb, watching myself wince in the bathroom mirror. Then she rolled still-damp strands of hair onto squishy, pink, foam curlers, which would surround the back of my neck until morning. I tucked them in between my ears and shoulders to sleep. Mama unwound my curls before Sunday school.

"Why can't we cut our hair, Mama?" I asked, squinting against the eye-watering yank of hair caught in the plastic curler clip.

"The Bible says that a woman's hair is her glory. Cutting it would not glorify God," she explained matter-of-factly, as she brushed my hair into shining brown loop-de-loops that bounced down my back, and plastered any wayward strays with fruity, plastic-smelling Dip-i-de-doo gel. "You want to make Jesus happy, don't you?"

"Uh-huh," I responded as I touched the bluebird barrette at my temple and wished my hair was jet black and straight, like a Chinese girl. Mama settled my ringlets on my back with a satisfied smile and a pat. She walked over to my closet and pulled out my favorite dress, a frothy, floaty, pink cupcake of a dress with embroidered daisies and layers of sheer skirt, leftover from being the flower girl in someone's wedding. I was a flower girl practically every other week, and Mama made all the outfits herself.

"I think I'll have you wear this one today, Ronna," Mama decided, slipping it off the hanger and poising it above my head. "Raise your arms," she directed.

I lifted my arms so she could slide the silky fabric on without messing up my hair. She zipped me up without catching any hair in the zipper and resettled my curls. Mama was an expert.

"Mama, can I please wear my strawberry sandals?" I asked excitedly. I knew deep in my heart that my denim sandals with red, embroidered strawberries on the toes would look amazing with my pink dress. I had to wear my favorite dress and shoes together.

"No, your sandals don't go with this one. Wear your black Mary Janes," Mama negated.

"Please, Mama, pleeeeeeaaase," I begged. "They do go, they do!"

"No, Ronna. Put your black shoes on. I'll spank you if you argue with me,"

Mama warned as she walked out, leaving me to obey.

Mama made the rules about clothes because how I looked was important. She always looked perfect. Everyone at church knew we belonged with Daddy and he was a sharp dresser, too. Church people were watching, and so was God. Fury rose in my chest as I shoved my feet in those hateful Mary Janes and fastened the tiny buckles on the sides. *I guess those buckles are pretty cute,* I thought, *but my strawberries would be better.* I checked my face in the mirror to see how mad I looked and to feel sorry for myself.

I joined Mama in the kitchen where she was putting roast beef in the oven. Our special Sunday breakfast of mandarin oranges slices out of a can and frosted orange rolls out of a tube, the kind that pops open, was already on the table. I climbed into my vinyl highchair with the zoo animals on it. Our new dining set had come with four chairs, so I still sat in my old highchair without the tray. Susan and Karissa were already at the table sitting in regular chairs. Mama had set our places with tiny glass bowls of mandarin orange slices and little glass plates with one orange roll each. Sunday breakfast was the closest thing to junk food we ever ate, and I loved every bite.

Susan counted the orange slices in her bowl. "How many did you guys get?' she asked, leaning over to count Karissa's oranges, the curl of her dark brown ponytail swinging over her shoulder. "I got one more than you," she determined with a satisfied grin. "Because I'm oldest."

"No fair. Hey, Ronna, are you going to eat your middle? The middle of the roll is the worst part. I'll eat it for you. It's gross, you won't like it," Karissa wrangled, spooning mandarin orange syrup into her mouth, her green eyes wide with feigned innocence.

I shook my head and shoved the gooey center into my mouth before she could convince me to hand it over. Susan and Karissa finished breakfast first, piled their plates and bowls in the sink, and descended to their basement bedrooms to get dressed. We had to wash the dishes after dinner, but not after breakfast. I slid my plate up onto the counter above my head and opened the cupboard to throw away my napkin. My pinkie finger stuck in the cupboard door as it swung open, pinching it sharply. I let out a piercing wail of surprise and pain. Daddy charged into the kitchen in an instant, wearing his undershirt and trousers.

"For Pete's sake, I am trying to study my sermon! What is all the commotion?" he barked as he yanked me off my feet and over his knee, sitting down on a kitchen chair in one furious motion. He was doing the work of God, and I had interrupted.

My bladder's reaction was immediate. "I have to go to the bathroom, I have to go to the bathroom," I sobbed and kicked as Daddy paddled my behind with his hand over and over.

His anger subsided like a demon fleeing the sanctuary, and he sat me up on his knee. I smelled his hairspray and cologne as I snuffled while leaving a damp spot on his trouser leg and feeling misunderstood.

He noticed the spot on his pants when he lifted me to my feet. "She peed," he half-laughed to Mama, who did not say a word. Mama led me to my bedroom to change underwear in silence while Daddy hurried back to their bedroom to study. No one looked at my finger, so I stuck it in my mouth. I would try to remember to be quiet when I got hurt.

Despite the spanking, we were all ready to go right on time and piled into the family station wagon, dressed and curled, headed for Sunday school. I followed Susan and Karissa downstairs to the church basement and through the fellowship hall, which always smelled like damp socks, and joined my class in the first room to the right. We sang Jesus Loves Me and recited the Bible verse of the day until all the kids had it memorized. Then the Sunday school teacher read a story from a paper pamphlet about a boy who disobeyed his mother and got chased by a bull. The boy barely escaped with his life. Everyone looked at me when the teacher read the author's name. Mama was the author. I wasn't sure what to say, because I was surprised to learn Mama wrote stories and because I had never seen a bull in my life and, as far as I knew, neither had she.

We always got home from church right about noon. As soon as our station wagon pulled into the driveway, Susan and Karissa jumped out of the back seat, racing to be first for the Sunday paper which always came while we were gone. Inside was a four-page double spread of color comics, the Sunday funnies. Whoever got to the newspaper first got the funnies first. Susan snatched the rolled up newspaper off the front step as Daddy opened the door. Susan and Karissa ran into the house, jostling each other, and arguing in whispers. If they fought over the funnies, no one would be allowed to read them. Whoever came in second had to start with Parade Magazine. I climbed out of the middle of the back seat of the station wagon and walked inside with Mama. We were home. My mouth watered as the savory smell of pot roast filled my nose. Every Sunday after church the whole house smelled like pot roast with carrots and potatoes and gravy. It was my favorite, except for the carrots.

After lunch, Karissa disappeared to her bedroom while Susan studied for Bible quizzing, a contest with teams and buzzers and timers. Teenage participants memorized entire books of the Bible and tried to win by hitting the buzzer first and answering trivia questions correctly within ten seconds. Daddy started the Bible quizzing program for the youth group, and Susan was the best at it. The teams were memorizing the Book of John this time. Susan sat in the blue recliner in the living room, reciting verses.

"For God so loved the world, he gave his only begotten Son..." she rocked back and forth, "...that whosoever believeth in him should not perish, but have everlasting life..."

Faster and faster she rocked, her words in cadence with the movement of the chair, the pen in her hand digging an ink stain into the upholstered arm with each motion. Her dark brown eyes were focused behind the gleam of her cat eye glasses, her hair slicked straight back from her face in a tight, high ponytail.

"For God sent not his Son into the world to condemn the world; but that the world through him might be saved," she continued, never looking at the Bible in her lap.

Susan's memory was impressive. She had already memorized the Book of John. Mama and Daddy were proud of her. I did not think Bible quizzing seemed like any fun at all, except for the buzzers, but I was jealous of the way their faces beamed with pride as she chanted.

I observed that the funnies were free. I pulled them out of the newspaper pile on the floor of the family room and dragged the pages over to where our little black dog, Cuddles, sat curled obediently on her rug next to the sliding glass door. I tuned out Susan's recitations and flipped to Family Circus and Hagar the Horrible. I could relax until it was time to go back to church.

Chapter 4
Treasures of Darkness

I developed a deep need for forbidden, worldly things. My most prized possession was a big, gold ring encrusted with twenty-seven rhinestones from my grandma that I was allowed to wear when playing in the basement. I loved that ring with unholy desire. Once, a sinner got saved at camp meeting and turned over her entire collection of costume jewelry to Daddy as proof of her commitment to Jesus; three double-decker jewelry boxes crammed full of sparkle.

Daddy set the boxes on the dining room table and opened them up. Susan, Karissa, and I crowded around the velvet compartments of twinkling, beckoning baubles. I was momentarily ecstatic, practically salivating, envisioning hours of fabulous dress-up play.

"Can we keep it?" Karissa yelled, reaching out to touch an enormous flowered broach. "Pleeeeeeaaase?"

"Oh, wow! Look at that one!" Susan exclaimed, picking up a giant cocktail ring.

"Nooooo!" he laughed as he snapped the lids shut. He picked the cases up and swooped them away.

We each got to keep an empty box. I don't know what happened to the jewelry. My cravings grew for things I could not have: a plastic Oreo cookie necklace with a bite taken out of it on a leather cord, a white plastic Donnie and Marie Osmond lunchbox. I did not know who they were, but they looked cool. The short, flippy, feathered haircut of a girl at the mall, a Barry Manilow poster. I concocted a plan. When I was eighteen, I intended to backslide temporarily and have permanent eyeliner put on, get my hair cut up to my shoulders, and my bangs feathered. Then I planned to replace all of my dresses with pants, so I had nothing else to wear, or perhaps compromise with less sinful culottes. My daydream involved taking a considerable risk that the Rapture would not happen while I was backslidden. I pictured myself returning to church to repent the split second I had finished performing these despicable acts, slipping into the back row with the other sinners, looking worldly and cool and ashamed. My shiny, shoulder-length hair flip brushed my shoulders and sexy, black eyeliner shaded my downcast eyes as I asked for forgiveness. Even after my hair grew out, it would still have that cool, straight edge across the bottom, and the Farrah Fawcett bangs would last for a little while; the make-up a permanent reminder of my walk on the wild side.

One day in second grade, my classmate Tom's mother came to the door as I sat at the math table sniffing my freshly dittoed worksheet. As I swiveled to see her, my braid caught on the metal screws of the chair back, pulling out a few strands. My eyes watered at the sharp sensation. This happened all the time; I gave my braid a quick yank and flipped it over the back of the chair. My seat was always identifiable by the long hairs stuck in the screws. I stared at Tom's mother, thunderstruck by her appearance. She was tall with a blond pixie cut, green eyeshadow, pink frosted lipstick, and a green mini skirt. I did not know mothers could look like that. She was clearly sinful, but she looked so good. Not like Mama or anyone else I knew, in their dowdy dresses, unadorned faces, and buns. I watched in awe until she finished talking to the teacher and left. Something about that haircut and make-up burrowed deep into my brain and stuck.

A few weeks later, there was a special assembly in the gym for Girl Scouts and Brownies. I became caught up in the excitement of the uniforms they wore but paid no attention to the activities described. The girls giving the presentation wore red berets and red sashes with pins. I ran home with the parental consent form and shoved the crumpled paper across the kitchen table to Mama.

"Please, Mama, you start off as a Bluebird and then a Brownie and then a Girl Scout! Can I do it?" I begged, practically bursting, willing to do anything to get that little hat.

"No, Ronna," she responded calmly, setting the form aside and turning back to the stove. Her big Betty Crocker cookbook was spread out on the counter.

"Whyyyy?" I asked, crushed.

"This is not a church activity. It's worldly. We can't spend our time on things that don't bring us closer to God," Mama settled as she stirred the pot. She was making Gentleman's Delight, a yummy, gooey casserole of noodles, tuna, and cheese. It was my favorite except for the pimentos.

Arguing did not occur to me. There was a wooden paddle on top of the refrigerator and Mama was not hesitant to use it if she sensed rebellion, such as a sassy tone of voice or too many questions. I was more than a little afraid of being told to lay across the side of my bed, bottom up for easy spanking access. That thing hurt, in addition to being humiliating. I had seethed many hot tears into my Bambi bedspread, not realizing until many years later that the damp cartoon animals were from a movie. A braver soul or a sharper mind might have spoken up with a pointed question or two for Mama, but I was not that kid. The consequences of rebellion were apparent in our family.

Aunts and uncles and cousins were shunned for their lack of belief. They had been raised in the church and decided not to stay; they were backsliders and, if they did not come back to Jesus, were going to Hell after they died or after the Rapture, whichever came first. Those family members did not come around much, but their fate was frequently discussed. Later in life, I connected with some cousins and heard of the sting they felt at our rejection. Once, while writing a thank-you note to an unsaved relative for a Christmas gift, I added: P.S. I hope you get saved before it is too late. My horrified sisters told me not to say that, but I didn't understand why not. We wanted them to go to heaven with us. Their lack of salvation was dire. Shouldn't we do anything in our power to encourage them to come back to Jesus? The Rapture could happen any second and they were going to be left behind. Personally, I did not want to be unsaved, shunned, or spanked.

I wandered away from Mama and the kitchen, downstairs to my playhouse where I invented elaborate games of house, church, and school by the hour, just me and my baby dolls. Sometimes I spanked them if they misbehaved. I plopped Crissy, my favorite doll with red hair that grew, into her highchair and took my yellow plastic pitcher into the bathroom. When it was full of hot tap water, I poured "tea" into the matching cup, then poured the rest into the sink and opened the cupboard door to watch it drain into the rusty coffee can underneath. I wondered how full the container was and reached in, holding it by the very edge to avoid the sharpness of the rim. As I slid the can into the light, a big black spider scurried around inside. I shoved it back underneath the drain pipe and slammed the cupboard door shut.

Time to play church. I pulled out my double-sided chalkboard on a stand. This I loved. I listed, in order of hotness, all the teenage boys from church, first and last names. Mama came downstairs with a laundry basket under her arm and saw the list.

"What are you doing? Why are you writing all of those boys' names on your chalkboard?" she asked, sounding concerned.

"Those are all the cute boys," I said. *Obviously*, I thought.

"What? Oh for heaven's sake. Erase those right now, Ronna," she ordered with her eyebrows up, as she piled laundry into the washer.

I erased the list as fast as possible, as she marched back up the stairs, in case she was headed for the paddle on top of the refrigerator. I rolled out the canister vacuum cleaner and parked it next to my toy piano. The corrugated vacuum hose curved out of the metal tube at just the right height to be my personal microphone. I grabbed the tube and howled off-key into the curve of plastic hose, "It is joy unspeak-a-ble and full of glory, full of glory, full of glory. It is joy unspeakable and full of glory, oh, the half has never yet been tooooold."

The pretend spirit moved. I began to speak in tongues and dance around in circles, shaking my head to make my hair fly around.

"Loolooloo, lakalakalaka, klerkakadalkala," I garbled.

The basement door at the top of the stairs creaked open again. Mama appeared, leaning over from the top step to meet my eye, eyebrows raised all the way up into cornrows this time.

"Ronna, stop that! Pretending to speak in tongues is sacrilegious," she exclaimed, nonplussed at my disregard of the holy.

I yanked Crissy out of her highchair and beat her plastic bottom until my hand stung.

Adjacent to my playhouse were guest quarters for missionaries on furlough. Daddy was the Director of the Foreign Missions Department at the Headquarters of the United Pentecostal Church. Missionaries were Pentecostals called by God to tell people in other countries about Jesus. They went to wherever God said to go for four years at a time, to preach and build churches. Furlough happened when they came home to see family and raise funds for the next four years. Their first stop was Headquarters and the guest room in our basement. They came and went with stories and pictures; filling my head with images of other people and places. A few of them stood out.

The Stonemans spent many years in Africa. They spoke Swahili, which they used if I encroached into the guest quarters with my big, listening ears. Swahili was a fascinating language to hear, like music with kissing sounds thrown in. Brother Stoneman had kinky hair, a wide face, and smile to match. Tightly-bunned Sister Stoneman was stern, but not unkind. They taught African women to cover their bodies; to dress the way the Bible said you were supposed to. The African women put on the white tee shirts the Stonemans handed out for modesty but promptly cut holes in them for their breasts to hang through, so that their children could still nurse. Unfortunately, there were no pictures of this. The Stonemans loved Africa and the people there, even though they were there to save them from themselves and to teach shame. The requisite slideshow always showed sweating black men in long-sleeved shirts, ties, and trousers. Their faces glistened in the sun as they stood in a barren churchyard, in front of a cement block church sporting a UPC sign. I always thought they had taken something interesting and made it not.

Brother Presley, a natural entertainer, and storyteller visited from the Philippines. He had an ebullient personality and played our piano with gusto, making up songs as he went. When he made up a verse about me, the warmth of his personal spotlight created a glow that faded when his attention moved to one of my sisters. We all got a turn; Brother Presley was cool that way. He brought beautiful Philippine dolls in beaded dresses with shiny, black hair made of thread. And he couldn't ever drink orange soda because once, on a very hot and thirsty trip in the heart of the Philippines, he bought an orange soda from a roadside stand and got very sick.

Daddy often traveled to visit the missionaries and preach at churches all over the world. I remember when he returned from a long trip to Africa. Susan, Karissa, and I flew to greet him, tackling him all at once. He almost lost his balance as he tried to set his suitcase down and hug us all.

"What did you bring us? What did you bring us?" Susan and Karissa squealed. I squirmed in between them to wrap my arms around his leg. Daddy was home.

"Wait a minute," he laughed, as he attempted to extricate himself.

"Ewwwww, you STINK!" Susan howled.

"I smell like cigarettes from the airplane. The smoke gets in my clothes," Daddy explained, as Susan and Karissa ransacked his pockets. "Your souvenirs are in my suitcase, you know," he chuckled.

The unfamiliar stench clinging to his suit filled my nostrils, pungent and sour. Daddy peeled us off and took his suitcase to the bedroom, where he unloaded treasures of wooden carvings, copper figurines, and beaded gourds, most long since lost.

During my eighth summer, our family went on a six week trip to South America to visit missionaries there. Daddy was the celebrity preacher at every stop.

In Argentina, we stayed at the Christianson's house, missionaries in Buenos Aires where white cows that looked as big as buses strolled down the middle of stone streets. One evening all the adults went to a church service, leaving the children from both families home alone. While they were gone, we heard booming, explosions. The next day we drove through the streets and saw bombed out buildings; empty, gaping windows with black smoke on the walls. We fell silent as the car glided past the damage on our way to the airport. I did not know who bombed the buildings or why but was glad we were leaving.

In Brazil, Mama and Daddy went with the missionaries to a sacred park to watch a witch go into a trance and cast a spell. They returned shaken, having seen the work of the devil up close, in person. Locals who protested the presence of the missionaries left chicken feathers on their doorstep, evidence of a satanic ritual, a curse. Street-side voodoo shops sold painted devils and carved, wooden fists, the sight of which struck terror into my heart. This was irrefutable evidence of Satan. He was working hard to defeat us. I was glad to get out of there, too.

We ended in Quito, Ecuador, traveling by truck through the jungle and high into the mountains to a camp where a revival was being held. Daddy gave fiery sermons in stops and starts so the missionary could interpret his message. I had heard Daddy preach many times, but never with pauses. "Give your heart to Jesus!" he bellowed, then stopped speaking as the missionary imitated Daddy's tone of voice and repeated his words in the local language, while Daddy waited. They had a rhythm, Daddy and the missionary, trading sentences effortlessly, back and forth in cadence. Daddy grinned as he preached; he was having fun.

The open-air revival tent filled with native Ecuadorean highlanders, some adults were no taller than me. The women wore beautifully woven garments and beaded necklaces from shoulder to chin. I watched a small child walk up to his mother, reach into the loose neck of her blouse, and pull out her breast. He nursed standing up while she continued peeling an orange. This blew my mind. That was the first time I had ever seen a breast. I lived in a home with four females and had never seen a nipple other than my own eight-year-old ones.

The babies were so beautiful it hurt. So were the young men; brown skin, dancing eyes, black hair, easy smiles... I was lust-struck. The missionary's tall, blond daughter was engaged to a handsome Ecuadorean man, and I was unspeakably fascinated. There were communal tents for the families that came to the revival and in one, a baby was born. He was named Donald after Daddy. Locusts the size of ballpoint pens buzzed through the air. Revivalists ladled soup out of a metal barrel, a black liquid with unknown substances floated in it; the smell of rotten fruit permeated everything. I was relieved to find out we were not going to eat there.

"Mama, why are they allowed to wear jewelry?" I questioned, jealous of the piles of colorful beads the women wore.

"They don't know any better. They wouldn't understand," Mama dismissed.

On the day we drove away, I gazed out the window as the jungle dissipated, wondering how a rule of God's could be changed for other people. Either a rule was a rule, or it wasn't. It seemed to me that once the Ecuadoreans were told about Jesus, they should have to stop wearing necklaces. But I did not want them to have to stop. I wanted to be one of them. I wished I did not know any better and could wear beads up to my chin.

Chapter 5
Cornered

As time in Jackson went on, and adolescence approached, I learned to fly under Daddy's radar, listening to radio music in secret and hanging out with the students at Jackson College of Ministries. I was unaware of his mounting pressures. Daddy had turned the rapidly growing Bible school into a financial success. He and some of the other teachers encouraged students to interpret scripture for themselves. They did not teach the pat answers dictated by the stated philosophies of the United Pentecostal Church. Word was getting around, and ire was up. Pitchforks were being sharpened. Whispered rumors of liberalism were in the air, although I never heard them. Daddy's explosive temper grew, unpredictably triggered by any little thing; always there like a scary soundtrack in the background, but I did not know why.

One evening, while Mama was taking Susan and Karissa to youth group, I heard a strange thwacking noise coming from the family room and walked down the hall from my bedroom to investigate.

I turned the corner to see Daddy holding a mouse caught in a trap over the fireplace, intently watching its violent struggle with an amused smile on his face. The mouse's panicked attempt to escape the flames was causing the hideous noise as it rattled against the confines of the trap.

"STOP IT, STOP IT, STOP IT," I shrieked, unable to comprehend what I saw.

"Oh, calm down," Daddy sneered, but lowered the trap and took the mouse outside.

I do not know what he did to the mouse out there. Heart pounding, I went back to my bedroom and shut the door, putting thoughts of the mouse out of my mind, not thinking about my Daddy torturing animals with a smile. I did not know what it meant but recognized the abnormality of his actions.

His violent temper was familiar; I had felt his open hand collide forcefully with my face in quick bursts of rage, but this was frightening in a new way. Telling Mama did not occur to me, because she was powerless. No one could stop Daddy from doing anything or even tell him he was wrong. The mouse was a good reminder to be careful around him.

This was back in the days of 45 records, tiny discs that played a single radio hit. Somehow, even though listening to the radio was frowned upon, Susan and Karissa had managed to collect a small pile of non-Christian records. They had 45s by Andy Gibb, Rita Coolidge, Climax, Debbie Boone, John Denver; every word to every song embedded in our pubescent brains. On a rare outing to Metro Center Mall, I purchased my first 45 for one dollar, a song called *A Little Bit of Soap* by Nigel Olsson that had tantalizing lyrics about make-up. And also about kissing, but it was the powder and lipstick mentioned in the song that fascinated me most. *Soap* was my current obsession on the radio, which I listened to in Karissa's bedroom, hunkered down behind her bed with my ear plastered to her clock radio, the volume so low it could not be heard by Mama when she passed in the hall.

When I got home from the mall, I slipped my new record into the pile of my sisters' 45s in the cabinet stereo, an upholstered piece of furniture that took up one end of the family room.

Daddy found my transgression later that evening.

"Ronna, get in here," his command resounded down the hall.

I poked my head in the doorway to the family room, surprised to see the entire family seated, waiting for me.

"What is this?" he accused, holding up my precious 45 for all to see.

"Alittlebitasoap," I trembled, feeling my face go blank even as my color rose.

"Play it," he ordered as he flipped the disc in my direction, holding it out for me to retrieve. He leaned back in his upholstered rocker and cleared his throat, hands gripped the armrests, and his mouth set in anger.

Shakily, I threaded the adapter onto the metal turnstile, slipped the disc out of its paper sleeve, and onto the adapter props. I set the control knob to 45 and clicked the ON switch, then turned around to face my family. They all sat staring at me in silence, as the whir of the stereo coming to life filled the room. I heard my record plop onto the spinning plate, and the needle arm creak up and over. We remained silent and staring as the needle scratched its way into the album groove and *Soap's* first bouncy notes blurted into the air, belying the seriousness of the situation. I hardly dared to breathe as Nigel's plaintive voice filled the room.

After a few endless seconds, Daddy snapped in disgust, "Turn it off."

A lecture on the evils of secular music and my personal shortcomings for listening to such unholy crap followed as I stood silent and burning, all eyes on me. No one spoke, but Daddy.

Somehow I found the courage to point out that Susan and Karissa had records, too (yes, I sold them out; yes, they were mad). I never knew if he confiscated their 45s or not. He dismissed me from the room. I fled, fuming and humiliated. And furious.

Soon after, Jackson College of Ministries purchased a new facility, and our family relocated to the other side of town to live near it. We left Pecan Acres behind and moved into a glamorous low slung Southern-style white brick home, artistically landscaped with waving clusters of pampas grass. At night, a crystal chandelier sparkled through the front window and floodlights reflected off the gleaming brick. I wondered if we were rich. An intercom system with a built-in radio wired throughout the house became my most reliable source of secular music, which I had not given up. If I sat at the kitchen table in the chair closest to the radio, turned the intercom off and the volume down as low as it could go, I could get away with a few minutes of radio time before Mama caught me. The radio felt like a lifeline, the lyrics of pop hits were clues to the mysteries of the unreachable world outside of my own, and I listened every chance I got.

The new college campus needed dorms, so Daddy contracted an old friend from Idaho, George Anderson, to build them. George came for the summer to get the job done. He was a tall, quiet guy who came around our house a lot. Mama and Daddy had known him a long time.

There was always a familial expectation of participation in whatever was happening at the college, whether it was cleaning, collating papers or, in this case, helping out at the construction site. I was accustomed to being on campus and loved going there because when I wasn't working, I was free to wander.

The new dorms were nearing completion and Daddy had Mama bring me to the construction site one evening to clean. She took me into a shell of a dorm room at one end of the hall, wheeling a vacuum cleaner in front of us. The floors were still cement, and the windows were open holes in the walls, which allowed for a slight shuffle of the stifling Mississippi summer air.

"Here you go," Mama said, parking the vacuum in front of me. "Vacuum up the construction dust in all the dorm rooms until you get to the end of the hall. Then cross to the other side and do those, too."

"Ok," I agreed and flipped the motor on. My mind wandered as the smells of damp plaster and concrete filled my nose. The early evening light was beginning to fade, and the empty rooms were darkening. I poked the vacuum aimlessly around the floor, tuning out the roar of the motor. A sudden shadow shifted to my left and George appeared in the dim light. I had not heard him coming. His legs were so long he crossed the room in three steps. He strode up to me, too close. By the time I turned, he was bending over me from his great height.

"Do you like me?" he murmured.

"Huh? Yeah-" I responded, looking up, confused.

George was kissing me, his tongue darting in and out of my mouth.

Then he was gone. I stood, frozen, the vacuum still running in my hand. I looked down at my maroon cotton skirt and dirty ankle socks. I looked down at my puffy maroon and white checked blouse Mama sewed for me. I had hoped its loose fabric made me look like I had started to grow breasts, but it didn't, because I hadn't. Now, the matching outfit looked childish and silly. Sweat stretched under my arms and blossomed on the back of my neck under my stringy ponytail. I finished cleaning the floor, brain a blank buzz.

Later that night, I stood in Karissa's bedroom doorway while she got ready for bed. "George kissed me," I stated, watching her face.

"No, he didn't," she sneered, looking away.

If Karissa did not believe me, no one else would. I went to bed still feeling the strange thrust of George's tongue. Not too long after that Mama told me to stop hugging men who came to our house because it was inappropriate.

"Daddy and I have noticed that you hang on them. Don't be so affectionate," she lectured.

This answered the unformed question that still hung in the back of my mind. I knew George's kiss wasn't my fault, knew he had broken some unspoken adult code, but if I told Mama and Daddy about George, they would blame me. I was too friendly and had brought this on myself. This information fit together like puzzle pieces to create a clear message: do not speak. No one was going to protect me from George, but I could protect myself from blame. Mama added that someone at church had called me "sultry." She appeared to be appalled by this description, said it as an accusation, a concern, a fault. I thought it was the best thing I had ever heard about myself. *What a great word*, I thought, hoping it was true. *Sultry.*

Seventh grade began soon after. I enrolled at a large public junior high on Jackson's north side, an enormous change from the small neighborhood elementary school I had attended. After one day in this foreign land, I was transferred to an "alternative" charter school in downtown Jackson, where the teachers and principal, all from up north, had interesting ideas about education and did not shave their legs. I breathed a sigh of relief because I could see the alternative school would accommodate my utter lack of interest in academics. They let students read books in a bathtub full of pillows and create their own curriculum. *I should be able to hide out here with no problem* I thought with glee. *I'm not going to have to do anything.* Ready to check out at age twelve. Once in a while someone at school would ask me about the strange church they knew I attended.

"Don't you go to that big church with the light-up sign in front?" they asked.

"Not anymore. Used to," I lied, unwilling to admit a connection to it.

"What does that sign say?" they pressed further.

"I don't know," I shrugged. "I don't go there anymore," I lied again, knowing my appearance gave me away no matter what I said.

As I attended my downtown hippie enclave, Bible school students from all over the country filled the brand spanking new dormitories. JCM hosted banquets for the students at regular intervals throughout the school year; planning began right away. These events were pivotal dating opportunities for the college kids, like Holy Proms with new dresses and corsages and crushes and pictures. A banquet date might lead to a relationship which might end up in marriage ordained by God. Much gossip circulated about who was going with whom, who had been asked, who hadn't, and what to wear.

Susan and Karissa were old enough to go with dates, but I attended with Mama and Daddy. College events were my main social outlet, as I had no peer friends or activities of my own. I was as excited about JCM banquets as everyone else.

Getting ready for the party was an intensive process, requiring much more effort and planning than Sunday night services. On the big night, already dressed in my ruffled, polyester maxi, I labored with my curling iron in the bathroom, trying to get a ringlet just right. Despite several devoted minutes of sizzling that exhausted piece of hair, it refused to dangle according to my vision. I let out a squeal of exasperation, even though I knew vocalization was risky.

Daddy barreled down the hall in his undershirt and trousers. "Ronna! What on earth is that noise about?" he yelled.

"My hair isn't working right," I stammered, reddening with embarrassment at my outburst. I knew I shouldn't have made that sound.

"There is no excuse to get so upset about it. What is on your face?" Daddy demanded.

"What? Nothing?" I said, turning redder, heart pounding now.

"Rae!" he screamed. Mama scurried in.

"Scrub Ronna's face. Get a wet washrag and wipe her face off. She is wearing make-up," Daddy ordered.

Mama dampened a washcloth under the faucet and obediently and firmly scrubbed my burning cheeks. She lifted the clean, white cloth to the light and showed it to Daddy, shaking her head.

"Hmpf. Okay," his anger ebbed.

"Do you wear anything on your face?" he interrogated.

"Just powder," I mumbled, handing over my colorless Cover Girl compact, designed for soaking up adolescent T-zone grease.

Daddy glanced at it and tossed it onto the counter. "Hmm, I don't know. I'll leave that up to your mom."

He stalked out of the room. Mama followed him without a glance in my direction. I tucked my compact into my purse and unplugged the curling iron. My errant curl did not matter anymore.

I began to hang out at the Bible school more and more after that, where

I could avoid Daddy and Mama, and for something to do. Eavesdropping on the conversations of eighteen and nineteen-year-olds, I learned titillating things, heard scandalous gossip, and began to wear padded bras and high heels. I also started making out with eighteen-year-old boys, even though I wasn't old enough to date them. At least at the college, people would talk to me, and I learned to kiss. Well.

Chapter 6
Lost years

A nineteen-year-old college student named Alan wanted to be my first lover before I left Jackson for Portland, Oregon. I was fourteen. Formal good-byes to my family had already been announced, so Mom and Dad stayed home from church on our last Sunday night in Jackson. The Bible school librarian offered me a ride, and I decided to go to one last service. I wore my sexiest black dress, teetering black ankle strap heels, and was feeling pretty full of myself. My frazzled hair was hot-rollered and hair-sprayed into submission, my eyelashes Vaselined and curled, and I was without supervision.

I sat by Alan at the back of the church where the reprobates and uncommitted lingered. Sitting in the back indicated you were not serious about church or had arrived late, which was the same thing. I posed, legs crossed, skirt pulled over kneecap-but just barely, forearm wedged across my non-existent tummy roll; wet with desire at Alan's proximity. He slipped me a note.

"You're beautiful," the scrap of paper said. "I want you."

"I want you, too," I wrote back.

"Are you ready?" he scribbled.

"I'm ready," I responded, pretending to know what he meant. "Scared of getting caught, though."

Dad had a way of knowing things and going too far with this boy would provoke a level of anger and punishment as yet unseen. Alan did not hold my hand. He always seemed to want to make out with me, but he did not want to be my boyfriend. I did not know how he felt.

I wandered around after the service, disconnected and done with the place. And already forgotten.

"I thought you moved," someone commented.

"Leaving Saturday," I said, hearing the dismissal in their words.

Alan told the librarian that he was happy to take me home. My house was on his way, no problem. She hesitated for a moment, then agreed. I did not realize what had transpired until I was in the car with Alan, driving down the dark, empty road toward my neighborhood, *Night Moves* on the radio. We were alone. No one knew where I was. I had no curfew. I felt worried. Had this happened by accident or had he arranged it? What was happening? My stomach tightened in a confusing mix of excitement and fear. Mostly fear.

He has no idea how much trouble I am going to be in if Dad ever finds out he gave me a ride, I thought. The repercussions of a transgression this severe were unimaginable. As we approached the left turn to my street, Alan drove past and turned right instead, parking under a street lamp. He leaned over and kissed me. Alan had kissed me before. The world dissolved whenever he did. Suddenly, Alan was in the back seat, and so was I. I laid across his body, wanting to be kissed, but not knowing what else to want. He rubbed my crotch with his hand, and I realized I could go no further. I had not considered taking off my clothes. My underwear was impossible to explain. I was wearing church clothes; underneath my little black dress were layers of manipulation that I could not allow to be seen. There was a half-slip to keep my dress from clinging to my pantyhose, a girdle to keep the pantyhose up, the pantyhose itself, and, in my granny-style underwear, a panty liner to soak up my constant adolescent wetness. All of these embarrassing items were going to end up wadded in a ball on the floor mat, and I could not bear that humiliation. Although, if Dad found out Alan had driven me home alone, it wouldn't matter if I had exposed my panty liner or not, we would both be dead. Paralyzing fear doused any lurking desire.

"Take me home," I insisted, panicking, practically throwing myself back into the front seat. And he did. Just as well, since I knew nothing about birth control.

When Alan dropped me off, I wiped the guilt from my face, straightened my slip and dress, and eased in the back door. My hair hadn't moved, of course.

No parents in sight.

So far, so good.

"Hi, Honey," Mom called from the master bedroom.

I jumped.

"Hi," I called back, forcing myself to stroll calmly to my bedroom and softly close the door. Moving into hyper-speed, I peeled off my layers of clothing, pulled on pajamas, and dove into bed. Whew.

I gradually relaxed under the covers, wondering what would have happened if I had stayed in the back seat with Alan, but was relieved to not have been caught.

Saturday rolled around. Mom and Dad drove their car, packed to the brim with everything required for a one-way cross-country road trip. Susan had married a couple of years before and moved away, so it was just the four of us in a two car caravan. I rode with Karissa in her orange T-Bird, crammed with every last bit of stuff that did not make it onto the moving van. My secret collection of sin music record albums were in a sliding pile on the floor behind the driver's seat. Some of them did not make it all the way. I lost Michael McDonald's *If That's What It Takes* and several K-Tel albums, warped by the heat of the summer sun baking the back seat. I never got over their loss.

We pulled out early and hit the road, driving all day, and stopping in roadside hotels at night. There were no stops to socialize, no preaching on the way. When Dad had somewhere to be, making good time was required. Karissa was somber and quiet. She left behind a boyfriend and a social life. While I was hesitant about the whole thing, there wasn't anything in Jackson for me to miss, except familiarity, and nothing in Portland to be excited about, so far as I knew. Before school let out in the spring, I pulled down the roller map of the United States, tracing my finger across the colored blocks of states, Mississippi to Oregon. So far away.

I wasn't old enough to drive, so could not help Karissa maneuver the T-Bird cross country. We listened to music on 8-track cassettes, and I slept a lot. During one afternoon nap, sun shining in the window, I dreamed as an adolescent in the throes of hormonal surging does. The longing for something still mysterious infiltrated my dozing.

"I know what sex feels like," I announced to Karissa upon waking.

"No, you don't," she answered.

I turned my gaze to the passing landscape and thought about Alan. *I want to know*, I thought.

We pulled into the parking lot of Conquerors Bible College in Portland, Oregon, mid-afternoon on the fifth day. Karissa sat behind the wheel staring at the ancient, institutional building that was to become our home. I looked over to see tears rolling down her cheeks as she gazed up at the sign on the bricks. I tried to work up a few tears in solidarity. The future did seem grim. We had arrived, though, might as well get out of the car.

We followed Mom and Dad through double front doors into a vast marble hall, the entrance to a circular complex of offices, classrooms, dormitories, and apartments, located next to the docks of the Port of Portland. Being summer, the entire place was deserted and silent. The administrative offices, including Dad's, were front and center. We followed him to the right, down the hall to the last door before the first breezeway. Our footsteps echoed on the marble floors. He opened the unmarked door, and we entered a three bedroom apartment right off the main hall. I had never lived in an apartment before, nor had our family ever lived on campus.

Most of our stuff must have gone to storage, but our beds, a couch, and dining set found their way into the apartment. Our dog went to live at our grandparents' house. Dad reassured Karissa and me that this living arrangement was temporary. We would get a real house and get our dog back soon.

Dad went to work in the CBC office, and I went to ninth grade in an inner-city high school on the bad side of Portland. Roosevelt High School might as well have been Mars, it was so different from anything I had ever experienced. Vicious, hard-eyed girls in rocker tees and black eyeliner stalked the halls. Lanky, long-haired boys obsessed with AC/DC slumped against the lockers. Whispered rumors of kids known to be pimps and prostitutes traveled behind them, as they strutted past. Couples made out in the back stairwell.

In my first class, a couple of girls seemed to want to be friends.

"I like her sweater," Annie whispered across the aisle to Nora.

"Meh, it's cheap, though," Nora grunted, not trying to not be heard.

"Yeahhhh," Annie continued, pivoting her opinion to agree. She turned a discerning eye to my fuchsia cowboy boots.

"I like your boots," she offered.

"Thanks," I gulped, cringing in my cheap sweater.

"Yeah, I like your boots, too," Nora conceded with a small nod.

Pecking order established, conversations continued over the following days, and I gradually relaxed in their presence. Thankfully, no school buses stopped at the docks, so Mom drove me every day. I asked her to drop me off five minutes earlier in the mornings so I could talk to my new friends before class.

"I don't know about that. I'll have to ask your dad," Mom considered soberly.

Mom submitted my request to Dad, and the verdict was handed back down the next morning. I already knew the answer. No, they did not want me to hang out in the halls of Roosevelt High School or associate with those bad influence kids, not even for five minutes before class. I was forbidden from having friends at school. I knew I wouldn't get another chance to not be the weirdest, loneliest kid in the place. There was nowhere else to go. To be fair, none of those kids had easy lives either, and they continued to be friendly, however, when social participation is forbidden there are limits to relationships, and they drifted away.

We went to a new church, a small, quiet, low-key kind of place, across the Columbia River in Vancouver, Washington. The music was vastly different from Jackson; no trumpet sections, no thumping bass, no black gospel influence. It was church without the show; soft, mellow, and snoozy. Our family walked in without fanfare and took our seats. After opening hymns, we were invited to the platform to be introduced, on a much smaller pedestal this time. The photographic proof of the moment shows Mom and Dad gazing at each other with smiles of satisfaction as Karissa and I glared stonily at the camera, furious and miserable.

The charismatic Christian movement was in full swing in the Pacific Northwest. Hypnotic praise chants replaced traditional hymns and frenetic rapture music. Lyrics were posted on overhead machines so the congregation could follow along while swaying back and forth to the simple plunks and strums of piano and guitar.

I love Thee, I love Thee,
I love Thee, dear Lord
We love Thee, We love Thee
We love Thee, dear Lord...

The worshippers appeared to be swept away, riding an invisible wave of sap. They were feeling something I wasn't, and I felt like the only sober person in the room. Detachment was not new, but in Jackson the cranking gospel tunes kept me awake and entertained, along with the task of keeping track of who was going out with whom, which couples had broken up between altar call and prayer room, and who appeared to be the hottest of them all at any given moment. Being forced to sing sedating hymns with lyrics of false truths based on intangibles that utterly escaped me, rage began to grow. Rage at being forced to sit-stand, sit-stand, forced to pretend, to never have a voice. The only acceptability was compliance, being an example, but now it was boring. I hated it all with the white-hot contempt of a teenager.

Soon after settling in, I started a part-time job in the kitchen of a nursing home called Harvest Homes, right around the corner from the college campus. I was comfortable there, pouring juice and washing dishes. One Saturday afternoon, a resident shuffled into the kitchen as I was setting tables for dinner.

"I think my roommate needs some help," she said worriedly.

I followed her down the hall to see a new resident whose name no one knew yet, sitting on her in-room portable toilet, cackling with glee. A steaming pile of feces spread across the floor.

"Hoo hoo hoo hoo hoo," the new resident was cracking up.

I was relieved this clean-up did not fall under my job description and headed back to the housekeeping office to report. While not a dream job, perhaps, Harvest Homes gave me somewhere to be and people to interact with; an escape. My hours, at $3.35 per, started after school through dinnertime and occasional weekends. The owners of Harvest Homes were old friends of my parents from way back, and while they were not real Pentecostals (Linda wore makeup and had frosted hair with bangs), I thought they would understand that I couldn't work on Sundays. After a few months of employment, my schedule included Sunday lunches more often than not, directly interfering with the Pacific Northwest Pentecostal afternoon church service, instead of the Southern tradition of two services, morning and evening. Pacific Northwest Pentecostals were progressive.

After a few missed church services, Dad shook my work schedule at me and slapped it onto the kitchen table.

"You are doing this on purpose. You asked Linda to schedule you on Sundays, so you don't have to go to church," he charged.

"No, I did not," I defended, shocked at the accusation. I never tried to get in trouble on purpose. That level of outright subterfuge had not occurred to me yet.

"Then you go over there right now and tell Linda that you cannot work on Sundays," he commanded.

I did so immediately, sweat rings staining my shirt as I explained the conflict. Linda looked a little surprised but never scheduled me on a Sunday afternoon again.

While the residents of Harvest Homes loved me and I loved them in return, I was desperate for connection with peers. And fun.

Then I met a boy from out of town named Dean.

I was nuts for that guy. We met at a revival and couldn't stop kissing, couldn't keep our hands off each other from the night we met. We wrote letters, exchanged pictures, and saw each other every chance we got.

His family came to town for a wedding. The parents attended alone. Dean and I had a perfect opportunity to be alone while our older siblings were distracted by each other. We wandered nonchalantly down the long marble hallway of the college without a plan that I was aware of. Dean tried the door to the central office. It was unlocked. No one was around. Without a word, we slipped in. Dad's office door was unlocked, as well. Our old orange and green striped velour couch was in there, transported from our living room in Jackson. We lay on the sofa, kissing in hurried silence. No pantyhose or complicated garments this time, just a purple string bikini that slipped out from underneath my denim skirt with ease, and that is when I lost my virginity. Searing pain and then something was over, but I wasn't quite sure what. A few drops of blood dripped into my underwear as I pulled them back on, while Dean searched the cushions for spots and opened the window a crack as if he had done this kind of thing before. Someone I know recently heard this story and paled. Turns out they still have that very couch. I am uncertain of its current fate. Perhaps it has been burned.

I'll never forget the next and last time I had sex with that boyfriend. His family was visiting again, another wedding perhaps. He and his brother were bunking in the empty dorm rooms, while his parents stayed in my apartment bedroom. Dean had broken up with me, and I was in shock. Breaking up meant I was damaged goods. No one would ever marry me now. I was like the white glove that had been dragged in the dirt. Sex was a contract; he was supposed to marry me.

Unaccepting, I snuck into his dorm room in the circle building and slipped into his sleeping bag in a desperate effort to remain visible. We fucked hurriedly. I heard the heavy outer door slam, Dad's pounding pissed off footsteps echoing down the hall. He was looking for me. His anger radiated through the walls, and my heart pounded against my chest. Dean and I stood frozen in the dark, not breathing, waiting for him to pass. As soon as the next door slammed, I ran like hell back to our apartment, ripped off my clothes, and jumped into bed beside Karissa. Dean's parents were asleep in my room and thank goodness for that.

Dad, foiled and furious, came into the room, shoved his face into mine and hissed, "Where have you been?"

"We were breaking up," I quaked, cowering under the covers.

"If we did not have company I would drag you out of this bed and beat the hell out of you," Dad snarled.

Things were going very badly for Dad at that point. He had arrived in a place he considered home to be among lifelong friends but instead found himself in a religious and political fight for his career. His desire to allow some free thought into this closed religious system whose basic tenant was to forbid free thought was a big mistake; his efforts misguided. Dad came under savage attack from the ministers in power in Portland and was openly accused of liberalism, of encouraging students to think for themselves instead of giving them the required UPC-approved answers to theological questions, just as he had in Jackson. He was considered a threat, and justifiably so from a certain perspective, as many of his students ended up abandoning the United Pentecostal Church in later years. Intellectual thought was blasphemy, the kiss of death. He was alone and scared and hurt. And angry.

At the time, I did not know what was going on. No one talked to me about any of the internal drama or talked about it in front of me. Or maybe they did, it is entirely possible I wasn't listening. All I knew is that Dad's temper had a hair trigger now and Mom was more silent than ever.

Dad's liberalism did not extend to my hair, and I was sick of the constant fixing, curling, spraying, and barrettes. I hated the way it advertised my oddity. The long dowdy skirts were depressing enough, but I had never wanted anything as badly as I wanted a haircut and concocted a plan to get rid of some length. Electric rollers were the new Sunday curl makers; no one used old pink foam rollers anymore. Overuse of hot rollers was known to cause split ends and severe damage, so I began to put them in my hair every night at bedtime and slept on them all night. The hard plastic spikes and metal clips dug into my scalp, but if I positioned them just right, I could find a comfortable spot for my head and drift off. The effect began right away. Week by week, my hair broke off at the ends and shortened, inching its way up toward my shoulder blades. I made sure to never have my back to Dad.

The strands of broken hair around my face shortened as well, almost up to my chin, now. I looked in the mirror, pulling them straight, checking the length. As long as they would reach my barrettes, I was safe. Then one day, almost without thinking, I picked up a pair of scissors and snipped a few long strands to frame my face. They weren't quite bangs but were shorter than they had any right to be.

Dad came into my room. I was working out on the slanted sit-up bench he had brought home from somewhere and put in my bedroom. I had begun to gain weight quickly after our move to Portland. The bench was a subtle hint.

"What have you done?" he charged, leaning in toward me. "Did you cut your hair?"

His voice pulsed with fury.

"Just a little around the edges," I whispered, eyes wide, leaning back, my toes flexed rigidly under the sit-up board bar. Denial was impossible.

He shoved his face up to mine, jaw clenched and rippling, hazel eyes blazing. I should have been able to smell his hot breath on my skin and his aftershave, but my senses shut down, as they always did when his rage was this close.

"Go ahead, then, cut your hair if you don't give a damn about my career," Dad spat, trembling with hatred.

His wiry body tense from head to toe, he whirled around and stalked out, leaving me hanging from my shins, afraid to move. I had never heard him curse before. Guilt and fear vied with an underlying knowledge that this was not normal. I was fifteen years old. My hair could not possibly be responsible for the career of a grown man. But it was. I stared in the mirror at the frizzy curls framing my newly pudgy cheeks, wondering how this was real and how I would ever escape.

Mom all but vanished during that time. She taught classes and worked in the CBC library, moved through the apartment. Karissa had a job downtown and hung out with the college kids when she wasn't working. I stayed in my room, laying on the floor behind my bed with my head pressed to my stereo, listening to pirated cassette tapes of Samantha Sang and Leo Sayer. Every breathy word of every ballad pierced my heart and left me longing for the escape of true love. My sole interest had been my relationship with Dean, which I clung to with the love-struck insanity only a hormonal teenage girl can muster. The demise of that relationship left me near suicidal. That is not an unusual thing in an adolescent, however, coupled with the underlying belief that I was now unlovable, damaged, and dirty, I sunk into a depression that went unrecognized as such. The problem was my attitude, they said. I would be happy if I were a better Christian if I prayed more, they said. Considering Dad's situation and my attitude, I am pretty sure I was a liability.

The valuable campus property by the docks was sold, and we moved across the river to an actual house in Vancouver, Washington with the Bible school housed in a rented strip mall. Soon after the move, female students wore snow pants on a sledding trip to Mt. Hood. They were seen by church people and reported to the CBC Board of Directors, the very men who were looking for a reason to get rid of Dad. Dad was confronted about this blatant sin of his students. When asked if he had given the women permission to wear snow pants in the snow, he admitted that he had. He defended his decision with the argument that allowing women to wear snow pants while sledding seemed much more modest than sledding in a skirt and that they were required to wear skirts while traveling to and from the mountain. They were also required to wear skirts over their snow pants after they arrived at the slopes. The board responded that any activity a woman could not engage in modestly in a skirt should not be done. Females could not play in the snow and honor God, and thus should stay home. The board and local pastors pushed Dad into a corner. They withdrew financial support from the college and discouraged Pentecostal families from sending their children to the renegade's school. The college was going broke. The snow pants debacle was the last straw.

Dad quit.

He left the only career and social circle he had ever known, left behind every friend he had ever had and he took Mom with him. They were no longer Pentecostals. They were alone.

I was thrilled because I thought I was finally on the fast track to cutting my hair off and wearing make-up, maybe even blue jeans. Maybe I could finally be normal. Things did not work that way, of course. Normalcy was not in the cards. My anticipation of freedom left no room for empathy for my parents.

Tenth grade started at my second high school, this time in Vancouver, knowing no one and starting over again. I went to school, did my work, at least the parts that were easy, and kept to myself. I snuck a book into the hard classes and tuned out. This would be why I still don't know anything about physics. Living in silence, working shifts at Baskin-Robbins, I got fatter. I got so fat that Mom did not want to make me a cake for my sixteenth birthday. The hurt on my face changed her mind, so I got a cake and a hope chest full of kitchen things I would need when I got married someday and had a husband to cook for. Life was reduced to going through the motions and keeping my head down. And eating.

One night, while working at Baskin-Robbins, a scruffy-looking guy came in, holding eye contact with me from the door to the counter. As he approached, I saw that his dick hung out of his open fly. He held my gaze as he ordered a Rocky Road cone, his smirk told me he was waiting for my reaction. I pretended not to notice, handed him his cone, and took his money. My lack of reaction strikes me as very odd now. I told Dad about it, but he said the guy probably did not realize his fly was open. I knew that wasn't true. He was wearing button fly jeans. I wanted Dad to be outraged, to bristle with protectiveness of me. But he did not. At sixteen, I had already learned to go blank. Telling Dad was a test, his response an affirmation that I should remain so.

Around about this time Dad started stealing my money. I saved almost every dollar I made, always plotting an escape, perhaps a one-way bus ticket to Florida. Or a backpacking trip around Europe. Every daydream ended with Dad calling the police, dragging me back home by my hair, and imprisoning me forever. I was too much of a realist for adventure, but I saved for it anyway.

Dad's name was on my bank account, and one day my money was gone, a thousand dollars, saved $3.35 at a time. I stood in the hall behind him, a safe distance away, as he tied his tie in the mirror on his bedroom wall.

Shivering slightly, I said, "My money is gone from my bank account."

"I needed it to pay the landscaper," he dismissed. "I'll pay it back."

Hard eyes met mine in the mirror as he yanked his tie into a knot. "What do you want me to do, take out a loan from a bank and pay interest to some Catholic or some Jew?" he challenged.

I did not answer, turned away, crossed the hall into my bedroom, and shut the door behind me, wondering if he would burst in. The next day I went to the bank and opened a new account without his name on it. I did not tell anyone what I had done. He figured it out the next time he tried to withdraw my money. He was furious.

I was angry, too. Despite having followed the rules as a child, despite having gone along with all of the moves, never complaining about the new schools, the new towns, and new people to be an example for, acknowledgment never came. Don't step out of line was the message. I went for a walk around the neighborhood with a boy from the Bible college. He was too hot for me, so I put on the one necklace I owned for confidence, a little gold chain with three tiny gold balls that I had secretly purchased at Disney World years before. I had never worn it. We wandered the neighborhood streets in the tepid Vancouver sunshine, chatting innocently. I got caught.

"Where have you been?" Dad seethed when I walked in the front door, well before dinner time.

"Just on a walk," I replied warily, omitting that I had been with a boy.

He glared at me suspiciously.

"Take that necklace off," he snapped and walked away.

Mom and Dad had gone to some Christian parenting seminar thing where they were asked questions about their children, to test how well they knew me. They came home with a questionnaire.

"Who is your best friend? Carrie?" Dad asked.

"No, I haven't talked to her in over a year," I admitted, as my throat closed.

"Who are you friends with?" he pressed.

"Don't have any friends," I answered, holding my breath against sudden tears and the flicker of hope that they would reach out to me. Maybe they would see me. Dad cleared his throat and folded up the paper in his hand, dropping the subject. He did not pursue the conversation, and Mom did not say anything.

During the same period, I often disappeared on long walks alone, two or three hours at a time, and my absence was rarely noticed. One afternoon, I had been walking for several hours, meandering through unfamiliar neighborhoods. I came to an empty house with a For Sale sign. I wondered what was inside. The door was unlocked, so I eased it open. A dusty spiral staircase and funky yellow glass chandelier filled the entryway, but otherwise, the place appeared vacant. Just before I stepped in, I realized I was about to be alone in an empty house, and no one on earth knew where I was. My skin crawled with sudden fear, and I left, taking the most direct route back home. No one would know where to look for me if something happened. If anyone tried to find me.

Those three years in Portland and Vancouver are difficult to define. However, they set the stage for the next period of my life. I wanted nothing more than to be rescued from that place, but no one came.

Without the support of the UPC, the church and school floundered, and my parents were almost bankrupt. Dad got mad at Mom for taking government cheese. Also, he made a friend, a black gospel singer named James who started coming to our church and our house regularly. Then Dad got a job offer from an independent evangelical church in Sacramento, California, so we got ready to move again, the summer before my senior year of high school. Karissa and I were excited about moving to California. No more Pacific Northwest rain and the church there was not so rigid. Women wore whatever they wanted, cut their hair, wore make-up, and looked normal.

Teenagers went to movies. Everyone had a television. Just before we left, Dad sat Karissa and me down for a talk.

"Now, I know that the church in Sacramento is more liberal, but if you think you're going to move down there and start wearing jeans and makeup, you're mistaken."

Oh, for fuck's sake, I thought. We loaded up and headed south on Interstate 5. To this day, Mom bitterly recalls that the California state border guards confiscated her pie cherries because they had not stayed frozen in the cooler.

Chapter 7
Close Call

I found myself home alone on my eighteenth birthday, six weeks into a new town, knowing no one. We were in another new city in another new state, the third one in high school alone. I was dazed by the heat of Sacramento, sweating in my pantyhose and polyester, frizzy hair in a dowdy twist, looking like anything but a California girl.

As soon as we arrived, Karissa started work at a travel agency. Dad and Mom went to their jobs at the church as the assistant pastor and secretary duo. And I attempted to navigate the beginning of my senior year at Del Campo High.

The day everyone drove away leaving me overnight in an empty house was not long after school started. Karissa scored free tickets to Hawaii from the travel agency and decided to take Mom on vacation. Dad volunteered to drive them to the airport in San Francisco, a couple of hours away, and I assumed I would come, too. Mom and Karissa carried their suitcases into the garage. I could hear them chattering and opening the trunk through the open door. Then I heard Dad pick up his keys.

"Time to go?" I asked Dad, grabbing my purse as Mom and Karissa got in the car.

He turned to look at me with a surprised expression. "Oh, well... you should just stay here, Ronna. It's a long drive, and I'll stay overnight near the airport. I'll come home in the morning," he said decisively, though there was also something careful in his tone. "I'll see you tomorrow."

I stood disbelieving, as he shut the door to the garage behind him. I stood by the door, listening to the car pull out as the three of them left together. I kept standing there as the automatic garage door whirred closed, surprised to be abandoned on my birthday. Shocked, even. No one had asked me what

I would do while home alone. There was no one to spend the evening with. I stood by the garage door numb with rejection. I drifted through the house to my new bedroom and sat down on my tidily made bed. Blank white walls stared back at me. The emptiness and silence pulsed, suffocating me as they closed in.

They left. Empty hours stretched out in front of me. *If I sit in this fucking house by myself staring at the walls all night on my birthday, I am going to go bonkers,* I thought. I had a car, an orange Pinto wagon that ran most of the time, and I remembered the way to Casa Maria's Mexican Restaurant and Bar at Sunrise Mall. Also, I hadn't had sex in the three years since Dean dumped me. No one had touched me in all that time, not so much as a hug. I was starving for attention, with an unhinged need to feel someone else's skin. None of the California boys in Dad's new church were interested in me because I was fat and still dressed like a Pentecostal. My desire for contact boiled inside. My craving to be with someone, anyone, throbbed.

At dusk, I drove my trembling Pinto down the wide, open streets to Casa Maria's and pulled into a vast, almost empty, mall parking lot beneath a neon sign flashing a red sombrero. Without hesitation, I parked and walked in the double wooden doors.

The bar was to the immediate left of the entrance. The bartender glanced up, but before he could speak, the only guy sitting at the bar looked me up and down.

"Come here," he said, with a motion of his head.

I walked over, trancelike, and slid onto a barstool beside him without a word. I did not have a thought in my head.

The bartender looked a little nervous. "Do you have ID?" he asked.

"No," I said.

"Let's go," the guy on the barstool said. He was Hispanic, not much taller than me when we stood up, with bushy black hair, and a thin, sparse mustache. At least 30, maybe older. I couldn't tell.

I followed him out, glancing back over my shoulder as we went, noting the look of shock on the bartender's face. Outside, the guy hopped into my car without any discussion. I followed his directions to another bar but got carded again, so we left and cut to the chase. We climbed in the back of my Pinto wagon, leaving the hatchback up. I slipped off my shoes and slid my underwear off. He had not told me his name, nor did he ask mine. I had not spoken at all, other than to admit that I was not twenty-one. My mind buzzed blankly as I watched the scene unfold around me.

"Turn over," he said, taking charge immediately. Then he pushed my skirt up and fucked me from behind. Right there in the parking lot, as I stared out the back in silence. My mind detached and floated away as he entered me over and over. It did not hurt. I couldn't feel anything. I heard his whispered groans as he pumped into me, faster and faster. I did not want him there after a while, but I also did not have any great urgency for him to finish. I watched from outside my body.

After he came, I climbed out of the back of the Pinto, ducking to avoid the raised hatch, and stood outside in the parking lot in the soft evening air. Felt the warm breeze on my face. I pulled my underwear on while the guy peed on the asphalt. I watched his steaming stream of urine flow underneath my shoes, an ugly beige mesh peep-toe flat with a bow on the toe. I knew I would never wear those shoes again.

I pulled the hatch down and got into the driver's seat, as he climbed in on the other side so I could drive him back to the Casa Maria parking lot. We still did not speak. I pulled into an empty parking spot. He hopped out of my car and into his own.

"My name is Louie, don't forget," he called to me as he drove off, music blaring through his open window. Prince's voice trailed behind as his Camaro accelerated and sped away.

I drove straight home, navigating the empty streets in a daze, darkness swallowed the space outside. Back in my bedroom, I stared numbly at the undecorated walls again. The whole encounter hadn't even taken an hour, and I was still very much alone on my birthday. I did not inspect my body or take a shower or think about why I had walked out my door and had sex with the first stranger I saw. Nothing. I crawled into bed, curled up around myself, and drifted off to sleep in the silence.

Back in the 1980s, pregnancy tests were available only at doctors' offices, nothing of the kind was sold over the counter. I did not have a doctor or any money. Within days of my self-inflicted sex collision, I was panicked. I secretly searched the massive Sacramento area yellow pages for pregnancy clinics, then scoured the accompanying city maps to see if I could find them.

Webs of streets stretched for pages of indecipherable blurry grids. Then I saw an ad for a free pregnancy test at a nearby church. Filled with dread, I made an appointment for 1:00 the next afternoon, even though I had not missed a period yet.

The appointment was scheduled during the school day. Skipping school after lunch might have worked but if I got caught my plan would disintegrate. So I told Mom I wasn't feeling well and stayed home from school. The woman on the clinic phone had instructed me to bring a refrigerated urine sample. While Mom wasn't looking, I snuck a plastic tub with a lid out of the kitchen cupboard, one of the containers she used to store leftovers. I peed in the cup, but could not put it in the refrigerator, so I hid it in my closet. I worried that room temperature urine would not work for the pregnancy test, but a cup of pee in the refrigerator would be unexplainable. I had to chance it. At 12:45, I told Mom I was feeling better and that I was going to the library. I slipped out the garage door with my pee cup tucked in a brown paper lunch bag and stuffed into my purse, hoping the lid would hold.

As the garage door clanked open, I turned to see a heavily made-up Asian woman standing on the sidewalk. A bandana covered her hair, she wore false eyelashes, thick black eyeliner, and blue eyeshadow. I did not know where she came from. I had never seen her before.

"You know what means the word slut?" she accused, from her spot on the sidewalk.

I panicked and jerked my head back toward the door to the house to make sure Mom was not in earshot.

"No," I denied.

Then I dove into my car, slamming the door shut. *Who was she? How did she know?* I wondered. I had to get out of there.

I turned the key, revved the sputtering engine, and backed the Pinto out of the driveway as fast as I could, looking around frantically as I reversed into the street. The woman was gone. Not walking down the sidewalk, not in a neighboring yard. Vanished as suddenly as she appeared. Had she been a hallucination? Sweat rolled down my back as I drove out of the neighborhood, carefully holding my purse upright to not spill the pee inside.

I found the church and the clinic, turned in my pee cup to the woman behind the counter, who informed me that in exchange for the information I sought, I was required to watch a two-hour anti-abortion film. Of course, a free clinic in a church would have a catch. I should have known. I had no choice but to cooperate and resigned myself to a two-hour wait for my test results. I slumped on a metal folding chair at the end of an empty row, alone in a dark, chilly room. As soon as the film started, I realized I had seen it in a youth group program.

"I've seen this film before," I said, sticking my head out the door. *Thank goodness,* I thought. *Not even Mom would believe I was at the library for two hours.* I was determined to keep this entire situation under control.

"Oh, ok, well... your test results were negative. However, it's too soon to know for sure," she said with concern. "You could still be pregnant. Since you haven't missed a period yet, the test might not be accurate."

I nodded. I knew it was true and carried a deep, unsettling certainty that I was pregnant.

"Would you have an abortion if it turns out you are pregnant?" she asked as if another option existed.

"Yes," I confirmed and walked out into the glaring sunlight. *If I can just figure out where to get one.*

Almost a week later, before Wednesday evening Bible study, I leaned against the church's bathroom cubicle wall as twisting cramps contorted my body. I slid down the cold metal to a squat, silently sobbing, and trying to breathe, intense pain drove all coherent thought from my head. I could not see straight, much less wonder what was happening. After a few minutes, the pains subsided enough for me stand up and catch my breath while clutching the top of the toilet paper dispenser. I had never felt anything like that before. The pain was similar to period cramps, but times a million and with stabbing knives. I fled the church building and drove home, sweating and shaking. Mom was on her way out the door to go to service when I got there. I explained I wasn't feeling well, again-the only acceptable excuse to forgive the cardinal sin of missing a church service—and went straight to bed.

Hours later, the convulsions returned with a vengeance and yanked me awake in the middle of the night. Spasms seared and rocked my body so violently that I could feel it in my chest. I called out to Mom for help. Mom called Dad, who was out of town, to ask what to do. I heard her low, worried voice on the phone. He instructed her to take me to the nearest emergency room in Roseville.

I don't remember the drive or checking in. No questions, no exams, no x-rays later, I was sent home with a diagnosis of possible pneumonia and told to lay low for a couple of days.

One day later, stabbing cramps began again with terrifying force. Dad was back in town by then. I called him at work.

"I need you to come get me. Come get me. Please," I begged, my terror evident.

And he did.

Dad took me to a walk-in clinic on Sunrise Avenue, not too far from Casa Maria's, where I had met the guy in the bar. There were questions and x-rays this time. And a moment alone with the doctor.

"Is there a chance you might be pregnant?" he questioned tactfully.

I nodded, relieved. Finally, someone had asked the right question.

The doctor told Dad to take me straight to the emergency room, a different one this time, and he did. I was still dressed in my tattered, lime green sweats that I always wore to bed. I knew going to the emergency room had something to do with the doctor's question, but had no idea what. My mind had started to blank again.

I sat in a padded, vinyl chair in the imaging area of the hospital, waiting for my name to be called. Dad sat, elbows on knees, in the chair beside me, inspecting his fingernails, his jaw clenched.

"Is this the first time you've had sex?" he asked tersely, not looking at me.

"No," I whispered. "Remember Dean?" My breath caught on his name as my heart jumped with fear.

Dad's jaw rippled. He cleared his throat and pulled his fingernail clippers out of his pocket, and began to clean his nails. He did not say anything else, but his rage electrified the air around us.

I leaned back, resting my head on the sticky plastic chair, heart and lungs vying for space. Fear of the repercussions that would come after this medical emergency was over vibrated through my body.

Now he knew. I was not a virgin and hadn't been for a long time. I had done a terrible thing more than once and had gotten myself into real trouble now. I was inconvenient again. What would he do to me after this x-ray thing was over? His silent fury overwhelmed any concern for myself. Whatever was happening inside my body was secondary to my fear of him.

Someone called my name. I do not remember following them into the changing room or what they said after that. I swerved onto the bench, unable to approach the folded, white cotton robe beside me. Mirrors and hooks began a discombobulated swirl as my head spun. *I think I am supposed to put that robe on*, I thought.

The ultrasound technician came in to see if I was ready, but I could no longer stand or respond. She helped me up and onto a table in the adjacent room, placed a cold instrument on my lower abdomen, and turned to watch the screen. Instantly, she was on the phone, urgency in her voice; words I could not decipher. Her voice sounded far away. She looked far away, too, even though she must have been standing right beside me.

Moments later, gurney wheeling down a hallway, voices yelling, operating room, bright lights, scissors blades ripped through lime green terry cloth, masked faces loomed...

"Count backward..."

"100, 99, 98..."

Recovery room. Slide from the gurney to the bed. *Really? So far away*.

The ultrasound technician stood at the foot of my bed, pale and shaken, surprised I had survived. Metal staples marched across my lower abdomen, a forever scar.

The nurse cracked, "You're gonna use birth control next time, aren't ya?" as she wiped me down with a wet sponge. My cheeks burned with humiliation.

"Yeah," I whispered into the pillow while she rubbed my ass.

"Your fallopian tube ruptured, ya know. It's called an ectopic pregnancy. You lost so much blood, you're lucky to be alive," the nurse remarked briskly as she hoisted the scrub tub under her arm and walked out, having delivered the only information I would ever receive about what had happened to my body.

I kept my face buried in the pillow. I had never heard of ectopic pregnancies or fallopian tubes before.

Dad stopped by the hospital once during my week-long stay. He half-sat on the edge of my bed as if he did not plan to stay long, then read scriptures to me, prayed, and left. Karissa came to see me every day after work, but Mom did not visit. No one mentioned Mom to me, and I did not ask where she was. I was relieved to not have to face her shock and disappointment. No one discussed what had happened to me that night, or who got me pregnant. No one asked me why or how I felt or what they could do or what I needed. No one yelled or cried or touched me. There was no conversation, just a big fat Holy Shit atmosphere.

What I did not know was that Dad had the family in communication lockdown. Karissa was forbidden to talk to Mom or anyone else about my pregnancy. Dad allowed Karissa to visit me in the hospital, but Mom was not allowed to come. Karissa thought that Mom did not know why I was hospitalized because that is what Dad told her. Years later, I discovered that Mom did know about my pregnancy, but Dad forbade her to talk to me about it. So she did not.

I never attempted to discuss my experience with anyone. This situation was all my own fault, and I knew I did not deserve comfort or forgiveness and I sure as hell did not want to hear another Bible verse. My scream for help was met with silence.

In the weeks and months to come, I floated away inside my head. I dreamed of a baby with velvet skin and deep brown eyes. My desperate reach for connection had backfired, and I had been punished, seemingly by God himself. Silent days surrounded me like a prison cell. No one spoke to me. I heard no voices.

This terrible thing happened to me
I did this terrible thing
My body is broken
I am broken
Please talk to me
Don't talk to me
Would it have been easier if I had died?
Would it?
A few weeks later, Dad sat at the head of the dining room table, papers

spread before him. The medical bills had arrived. He motioned me to a chair. I sat.

"Brother Mackey had to backdate the insurance paperwork to get this thing covered," he pronounced as he cleared his throat and straightened papers purposefully into stacks. "We have a $3,000 deductible. I think it's only fair that you pay it."

"Okay," I murmured.

"How much can you pay per month?" he asked, his mouth set.

"$150? I'll get a job," I promised.

"Mm. Ok." Dad accepted, returning his attention to the stacks.

Something had been bothering me, though. What happened would not have happened if I had been appropriately treated during the first trip to the emergency room. And my father was a stickler for justice.

"Dad?" I said cautiously, "Umm, I'm just wondering why you aren't suing the first hospital for negligence. They said I had pneumonia," I felt tremulous.

"I would have if something had happened. It was a close call," he said.

There could be no more complete proof of my personal irrelevance than that it did not matter if I died, beyond how he would handle the bills. Solid evidence that my emotional and physical state were of importance to no one. When I look back at all of this now, I am not quite sure how I survived, or if I did. What part of myself vanished during that time?

Six weeks absent from my senior year, no one noticed when I went back to school. I had been a new face, anyway. I limped through the rest of the school year, heavy with heartbreak, pretending the fabricated appendicitis story Dad told the church people was true.

Decades later, a therapist told me, "Find a picture of that teenage girl, from around the time of the tubal pregnancy, when you were alone, and your family was fractured. Every morning, look at her and say, 'You're with me. I've got you, and I am going to get you through this.'"

I did it. I found a picture of myself that I could hardly stand to look at, snapped at the lake with my family. I drove to meet them for a picnic in a panic, crying and pleading to God all way, *please don't let me be pregnant, please don't let me be pregnant*. Knowing I was, but with no idea what was coming. The young woman in the picture is hungover, fat, scared, and miserable and about to have a life-threatening event. Every morning for a month, I reached for that picture and gave her a good look until she met my eyes.

"You're with me," I said. "All day. I'm going to take care of you."

This self-compassion felt impossible at first but became easier as the days went by. We both started to believe I could take care of her. Somehow during that month, I began to look at that miserable girl in the photo with empathy, instead of shame and hatred. I pulled her toward me through the years, the first time she had ever not been pushed away.

Part Two

Chapter 8
Out

Dad arrived home the day after dropping Mom and Karissa off at the airport for their Hawaiian vacation, much later than he promised. I heard the car door slam. Then another door. Someone was with him. The front door burst open.

"Surprise! Look who's here!" Dad announced in a sing-song voice as if he was walking in the door with a birthday surprise.

Dad's friend, James followed him in, suitcase in hand. His black skin gleamed in the too-bright Sacramento sunlight streaming in around them. Dad knew James from Portland. I knew him, too, but I did not know they were close enough friends for him to show up unannounced 600 miles from home while Mom and Karissa were in Hawaii. The last time I saw James was when he sang a love song at my parents' twenty-fifth wedding anniversary party.

"Heyyy, girl, how are youuuu?" James greeted with his familiar smirk as he reached toward me with a one-armed, half-hearted hug.

"Umm, hi, fine, how're you?" I replied, trying not to show my surprise at his presence. *What is he doing here?* I thought.

Dad never inquired how I had kept myself entertained on my birthday the night before so I didn't bring it up. The three of us ate dinner together as if somehow this was normal and, later that evening at bedtime, James walked down the hall into my parents' bedroom and shut the door. I watched as the door closed behind him, leaving Dad to face me in the hallway.

"Isn't James going to stay in Karissa's room?" I asked in shock.

That was my parents' bedroom. The master bedroom. Where my parents slept together. I wasn't even allowed in there. Dad and I were both poised as if for flight outside our respective bedroom doors, each eager to disappear behind them.

As he turned away, Dad explained, "You know, it's just like when you have a friend over." His tone was conciliatory. *You understand*, the tone implied, *we're going to stay up late and gossip, maybe do each other's hair*. But I did not understand-I did not have friends to have over, and my insides screamed *how can you not see that I am always alone?* He opened his bedroom door and took a step to move in.

"Oh," I nodded and stepped into my bedroom, too, shutting the door behind me. I tried not to imagine what was happening behind the other door. I did not know what was going on. Except maybe I did.

No one mentioned James' visit after Mom and Karissa came home. A few months later, not long after my tubal pregnancy debacle, someone saw Dad at a gay bathhouse in downtown Sacramento. They informed the pastor, who secretly fired Dad. I did not know about the bathhouse or the firing, I only knew suddenly Dad moved to Los Angeles. For work, he said. Things weren't working out for him at the church. His longstanding policy of nobody talks to anybody about anything unless I say so was in full effect. The story about relocating by choice was the explanation given to the congregation; his resignation letter was read from the pulpit after Dad was already gone. The same story was told to us all, including Mom. No one told her the real reason Dad no longer had a job as the assistant pastor, even though she was still the church secretary. No one told her that he was caught with his dick in a glory-hole or whatever. Dad certainly did not tell her. He just left, leaving us all to fend for ourselves in the dark.

Dad found employment selling insurance in L.A. and James joined him there. Preaching and selling insurance struck me as similar lines of work. I figured he would be good at it. Mom was left alone, trying to make ends meet. She believed Dad's lies that this separation was temporary, that they would continue his ministry somewhere else; that James was just a roommate. Dad had always been honest with her, brutally so.

One evening, Mom brought up my apparent lack of devotion to God, again. I no longer attended church services as there was no one with the power to force me. My disinterest was a consistent aggravation of hers.

"Where is Christ in your life, Ronna?" Mom started. "Your father and I are worried—"

"Mom, Dad is gay," I interrupted. "James slept in your bed with Dad while you were in Hawaii."

"He stayed in our room?" she responded as heartbreak spread across her face.

"Yes, Mom. Right in front of me. And now they live together. How long has it been since he slept with you?" I challenged, no longer willing to go along with their farce of a marriage.

"Not that long," she snapped.

"Then you should probably be tested for AIDS," I declared bluntly and walked out of the room. Tired of being considered the wayward one.

I was twenty-one years old when I moved into Whitney Arms apartments, an old two-story complex with a glittering swimming pool flanked by two towering palm trees which cast no shade over the baking concrete courtyard. The Whitney Arms vibe was derelict but quintessential, old-school California with dirty white adobe walls and wrought iron railings. Most of the residents appeared to be senior citizens. None of the less expensive studio apartments were available, so I rented a one bedroom for $185 per month, $75 more than I had planned to pay. The extra money would have to come out of my food budget, but I was thrilled at the prospect of living alone and would happily go hungry to do so.

Karissa and her husband, Gary, helped me haul my meager belongings into my new place. I had a mattress on the floor, Karissa's atrocious hand-me-down loveseat, a stunningly ugly lamp, and that was about it. The dishes, silverware, and set of pots and pans from my hope chest stocked the kitchen cupboards. One thirty dollar trip to the 99¢ Store provided a complete supply of cleaning products and kitchen utensils. After payday, I bought a card table and two folding chairs from Target and a big bottle of Tanqueray. It was fucking perfect.

Mom stopped by my apartment once before she left Sacramento for Washington State. She walked in with a smile, eager to see where I landed.

"It looks good. Cute," she said, patting my arm and smiling bravely.

"Thanks, Mom," I said, hoping she wouldn't stay long.

As we stood together in my mostly empty living room, she wrapped her arms around my shoulders and began to weep. I stood stiffly, wanting her to go. Thoughts of my own impending freedom superseded any appropriate empathy for what she faced; moving back to Vancouver alone with no income and an absentee husband. She was still waiting for Dad to be honest with her about their future together; still clinging to the old habit of letting him make the decisions. I couldn't wait to be away from their drama. After she left, I closed the door, and relief flooded my veins.

I learned to grocery shop on a dime right off the bat. My sixty dollar monthly food budget kept me in little packs of three dollar butterfish and fifty-nine cent heads of iceberg lettuce; whole wheat bread and skim milk for breakfast, and that was what I ate. I began to lose weight. I had never been happier if control is the same thing as happiness. There was a sense of safety within my own walls. After I settled in, I sent cards and wrote letters to my grandparents and aunts and uncles, but heard nothing in return. No one called or wrote back. No one knew my routine or came to visit. The realization occurred to me that if I died in my bed, no one would come looking. I imagined being taken off the schedule at work and chalked up to "Fired-did not show up for shift." How much time would pass before someone found my body? The landlord would come looking when rent was due; otherwise, I no longer existed.

I worked long hours to support myself, learning restaurant bookkeeping and lower level management. The restaurant office was not much more than a broom closet adjacent to the cacophony of the kitchen which cranked out an endless stream of burritos and burgers; steam and grease thick in the air. Careful navigation over sticky floor mats on slanting floors was required to get in and out of my broom closet office. Weekend night shifts were long and late. Karaoke wrapped up at midnight, and the bar closed at 1:00 am. The deposit had to be counted and dropped into the safe in time to walk out to the parking lot with the last bartender, for safety. He kindly checked the back seat of my car before I opened the door, which informed me that I was in more danger than I had realized. His moment of thoughtfulness felt like the warmth of the sun and made me want to sleep with him.

One Sunday morning, while arriving with the breakfast crew at 6:00 am, I unlocked the back door to the kitchen. Two of the cleaning crew guys were handcuffed facedown to the ice machine on the tiled floor, in a puddle of leaking ice water. One of them tried to yell through the gag in his mouth. I did not know if whoever had tied them up was still in the building. I whirled around and ran back to the parking lot to tell the incoming cooks, then ran next door to the fire station for help. I pounded and pounded on the fire station doors, but no one answered. After a few minutes, I gave up and ran back over to the restaurant where the cooks had rescued the cleaning guys and called the police from the office phone. The cleaning crew was okay and had already gone home. The police did not need a statement from me. The safe at the back of the office had proven impenetrable, the burglars had only managed to scratch the surface around the keyhole. I looked around for someone to talk to about it, but the cooks were already prepping for lunch. There was nothing to do but get to work myself. I opened up the scratched safe, pulled out Saturday night's deposit, turned on the radio, and got to it, alone.

Despite being surrounded by people my own age, I found it difficult to connect with anyone. I drank to excess and slept around. Everyone else was doing the same, but somehow I wasn't doing it right. They seemed to be having fun and being cool, but I wasn't.

One of the cocktail waitresses invited me to see the movie *Die Hard* on a Saturday afternoon. I had only been to a movie theater a couple of times. I did not understand the point of this film; it did not make me want to see more movies. I drew the line when she invited me to see the rock band Rush in concert. I hated the disconsonant noise of hard rock. I had spent the last ten years listening to Barry Manilow, Air Supply and old-school country artists like Merle Haggard and George Jones. John Cougar Mellencamp was about as rock and roll as I could handle. I had developed a deep love of R&B and listened to Motown, Marvin Gaye, and Michael Jackson, the familiar rhythms a reflection of my Southern gospel roots. My inability to participate in the activities of my peers left me unable to accept friendships when they were offered, and my tendency to get drunk as quickly as possible made me an unpleasant companion.

I never had an extra penny, and definitely had no money for drugs, which scared me anyway. Most of my clothing was left over from high school and church days. Anything I acquired since then had a decidedly slutty vibe, black patent leather spiked heel witch boots, tight skirts, and skimpy tank tops, combined with frumpy church dresses and cotton blouses from the old days. A young woman from the restaurant took me along to the mall one afternoon. I followed her into a shop of subdued grown-up clothes. I watched, fascinated and a little repulsed, as she purchased a pair of slacks, a matching blouse, and earrings, for no reason other than she wanted them. She plunked down thirty dollars and walked out with a self-satisfied smile, shopping bag swinging from her hand. Who had an extra thirty dollars for clothing? Why would anyone buy something so unsexy?

My hair was a conundrum. Regular cuts were out of the question, but my curls disguised the neglect. Amateurish attempts with cosmetics were haphazard at best. I was a mess. I still had a tendency to go on long walks with no destination which helped keep me in shape, along with the constant scarcity of food. I had a sense of detachment regarding my physical self. I couldn't tell if I was overweight or not, if my clothes fit, or if I was attractive. I was always surprised to hear that I was thought to be odd because I assumed people couldn't see me. When you feel invisible, it is difficult to track the consequences of your actions or see how your actions affect others. I did not know what I was doing wrong or how to be normal. I did not know how to be with people sober. The only sensation I could feel was sexual. Being touched, even by a stranger, was better than the screaming aloneness of living in my skin. The physical contact available to me was to offer my body. So I did.

Deep into a Saturday night, a singer who performed at the bar kissed me on an alcohol and performance fueled whim as he walked by my bar stool. Martin was tall, lean, and muscular, with a voice and face like a freckled Lionel Ritchie. His kiss set my lower soul ablaze. We had instant, electric sexual chemistry and stared at each other in astonishment as he walked back to the stage.

He took me to El Torito's for drinks a few nights later. I wore my favorite, super-soft, deep purple sweater, sure that it was flattering and irresistible to touch. The sweater was a risky choice, however, because it could not be machine washed and might smell of reconstituted body odor if I got too warm. We sat in a booth by the dance floor sipping gin and tonics while I worried about what smell dancing might instigate. Martin was kind of an asshole, aloof and uncommunicative but there I was on a real date with a hot guy, so I acted like I did not notice. I hadn't been on many dates and wasn't sure how men behaved in that scenario. I figured I was doing something wrong. I listened attentively while he complained about his aching knees.

"Gee, I'm sorry you're in so much pain. Are you okay?" I asked with concern, unsure why we were planning to dance.

Martin rolled his eyes.

"Alright, MOM," he retorted and got up. "Let's dance!"

I followed him onto the dance floor in confusion, embarrassed by his sarcasm. We left after a couple of songs. He kissed me in the parking lot, standing in between our cars. The sexual chemistry of the first kiss was still there. I melted from armpits to knees. I might not have had too many dates, but I had had a lot of kisses. This had never happened to me before. He begged me to come back to his place and despite my desire do so, I was scheduled to work the opening shift at 6:00 am. Nothing but nothing got in the way of work. If I did not work, I was homeless. Missing a shift was not an option. There was no safety net, no plan b, nowhere to go. My personal financial safety was the one line that could not be crossed; the one boundary I was willing to set to protect myself. Everything else was up for grabs. I put Martin off, but not for long.

A few nights later I was at his place, Marvin Gaye on the stereo. Martin sang *Sexual Healing* to me as he laid me back on his bed and rolled on a condom. His penis was so big, penetration was painful for the first time since the first time. I felt alive and real. The numbness I lived in melted away as his enormous cock stretched me to capacity. I was hooked. We lost his condom. I found it later, stuck in the only place it could be.

Martin never took me out on another date. We immediately had a sex-only relationship. He would not speak to me at the restaurant; did not want to be seen as my boyfriend or even as my friend. We were not dating. I was hurt by his treatment but did not understand it and so pretended it wasn't happening. Rejecting him in return did not occur to me as if somehow I did not have the option of telling him to fuck off. I told myself I loved him, a pattern of chasing rejection that would remain in place for decades. Martin was the one person who did not feel like a stranger, and I could not face being completely untethered. I was willing to put up with any treatment in exchange for feeling alive in his arms.

One night, late, he called and invited me over. I went, of course. We had a glass of wine and began kissing. I stood on the couch to match his height. His mouth opened under mine and I opened my lips, letting Fume Blanc run onto his tongue. He grabbed my body then abruptly let go. As I caught my balance on the edge of the couch, Martin turned around, bent over, and grabbed his head. He was visibly upset, leaving me standing on his couch with wine on my lips.

"What is wrong with you?" I asked, confused.

"I have a girlfriend!" he burst out.

"WHAT?" I sat. "For how long? All this time?" I wondered, my voice cracking.

"No! NO! I just started going out with her," he moaned, "but that thing you did with the wine was really sexy."

I set my glass down, picked up my keys, and ran. My car hurtled through the dark streets to my apartment, and I threw myself onto my shitty loveseat. The phone rang. I let it ring. He called again.

"What," I said flatly when I picked up the phone.

"I'm sorry," he said.

"You should have told me," I accused.

"I know, I'm sorry. I just can't say no to you," Martin admitted.

I couldn't resist his words or his desire. He wanted to come over. I did not tell him no. I opened the front door and returned to the couch, waiting, watching the moonlight on the palm trees.

He walked in, striding purposefully towards my bedroom. He did not see me on the couch, wrapped in a blanket.

"Hey, where ya going?" I spoke to get his attention.

He stopped and turned, dropped his jacket, and knelt in front of me, pulling me into his arms, peeled off the blanket, and devoured me on the floor. We did not make it to the bedroom. When Martin left, my downstairs neighbor pounded on her ceiling with a broomstick. The next day she asked me to be quieter.

"I could hear every breath," she snapped, disgusted. "Also, you left your laundry in the dryer again. I folded it. Again."

Martin did not stop seeing his new girlfriend, and I did not stop pining for him and calling at inappropriate hours. That someone could desire me so much but not want me still did not compute, even after all that miserable fucking. I could not understand that sexual desire did not hold emotional responsibility. He could fuck me and not want me. He could fuck me and not even like me.

Chapter 9
Blind Faith

We met when I was 22, and he was pushing 30. The fact that Roger had a minimum wage job as a courier and I was technically his boss should have given me pause, but it did not. We had a great time with after work drinks down at The Distillery, a dark dive in downtown Sacramento, a shared sense of humor, and a high degree of friendship chemistry. Roger was creative and hilarious; a sarcastic and entertaining loudmouth. He looked like a Viking. His blond hair shone like silk. Perfect, white teeth blazed behind full lips, and he had a barrel chest, thighs like redwoods, and a big laugh. He asked me about myself and listened to my story. No one had ever done that before. Our first date was an impromptu picnic lunch of goose liver pâté, brie, and baguette which Roger spread out on a table right in the middle of the office. We ate in front of our co-workers, who looked on in amusement, and then we took a stroll around the block. He kissed me, standing on the office steps, as a misty rain began to fall.

Later that afternoon, with love vibes pulsing in the air, Roger stood close to me, and asked, "What do you want?"

I knew what he meant. He was asking what I wanted for myself.

"I want to get married and have babies," I answered immediately, without looking up, holding back sudden tears from the sharpness of that desire. Roger caught his breath, turned away without a word, picked up his stack of deliveries, and walked out the door without looking back.

Well, now he knows, I thought, watching him exit. *He'll either be in, or he'll be out.*

On our second date, Roger took me to a fancy rooftop bar overlooking the lights of the Capitol. We sat at a polished wooden table with leather chairs that swiveled, ice clinked in tiny crystal glasses. Nearing the end of my second drink, I excused myself and went to the restroom. On a whim, while sitting on the toilet, I stuck my middle finger into my vaginal canal. Back at the table, I leaned toward Roger and, holding his gaze, softly slid my finger into his mouth without a word. His eyes widened, and he began to laugh. I smiled. We went back to my apartment soon after. It seemed like he could handle me. He hadn't run away from the idea of marriage and babies, nor was he shirking from my wild side. Maybe he would stick around.

Roger was a writer in his spare time and wanted to be a movie maker, as well. This courier thing was temporary because he was working on a script that was going to sell, for sure. I read it and believed him. He was good. Really good. The script was plotted out on storyboards with illustrations he drew himself. We went location scouting on the coast, and he introduced to me to his friends in the movie business, editors, and costume designers. There was no doubt Roger had a brilliant mind. Evenings after work, I lay on his couch reading scripts, howling with laughter, and falling in love. He loved that I loved his work.

Roger was my life raft. The thought never occurred to me that I could enjoy our relationship but wait for marriage and babies. Emotional needs were gnawing my gut. The lost pregnancy of my teens had broken my heart in a million ways, and I was still deeply shattered. Having a family of my own was the way to fill the holes in my heart. I did not know about therapy, or how much time I had to walk through the pain of my past. I did not realize how much understanding there was to gain. I did not feel like I had any time at all. I was in a hurry to find solid ground.

As the months went by, Roger and I had a lot of enthusiastically vanilla sex without exploring each other. We had sex on the couch, on the floor, and at lunchtime, never taking the time for foreplay. I was always ready and his touch always welcome. Our connection felt like love to me. I had no idea what treatment to expect in a partner, not in the opening doors for you kind of way, or in sharing the rent, or taking an interest in my pleasure. It seemed obvious to me that because we loved each other, we should get married. My need for babies and emotional security trumped every subverted logical thought. The fact that Roger moved into my apartment, but would not help pay the rent, that he would watch the latest Star Trek movie over and over, studying it with complete absorption, that he never had any money, I set aside. Roger agreed that my religious upbringing was nutty fruitcakes, so I felt understood and validated. It was enough that he talked to me. It was enough that he made me laugh. It was enough that he was there. For the first time, life did not feel tenuous.

We discussed marriage after a few months of living together. I needed a concrete plan to be sure he was serious. Roger said we would get engaged in August. I waited patiently for his proposal because I thought it was up to him. The man proposes, and the woman says yes, and then everything is settled.

I became anxious as August came and almost went. We wandered aimlessly through Lucky's grocery store on a sweltering Saturday afternoon, on the last day of the month. I appreciated the supermarket's air conditioning but was feeling at loose ends. He must be planning to propose tonight. *He hadn't forgotten, had he?* I thought as I stared at the produce piles with disinterest.

"I do not feel like cooking at all," I declared.

"Ugh, neither do I," Roger agreed.

We walked back out to the car empty-handed, through heat waves rising in noxious fumes from the sticky parking lot tar, laughing at our inability to make a dinner decision.

"Hong Kong Café sounds good," Roger suggested as we stood next to his Honda with the doors open, waiting for the blistering air inside to dissipate.

"Perfect! I'm starving, let's go," I said, relieved to have a plan. Time to get on with it. We were about to be engaged.

I had butterflies in my stomach as we drove down I Street to Broadway, unsure if he would come through. August was almost over, just hours left now.

Thirty minutes later, burrowed deep in a round red fake leather booth, surrounded by plates of steaming fried rice and chicken swimming in basil and garlic, conversation meandered without purpose. Ripped vinyl scratched the backs of my sweating knees. He wasn't getting to it. There did not seem to be anything on Roger's mind but eating.

"It's the last day of August," I pointed out, lifting my thighs, in turn, to unstick them from the seat.

"So it is," he chuckled and raised his eyebrows questioningly.

He had forgotten, but there was no way he was getting off the hook. He said August.

"I thought we were going to get engaged in August," I needled, my heart sinking with disappointment that I had to say it.

"Oh, right," he hesitated. "Well… then there is only one thing left to say. Will you marry me?" he asked softly, with a tentative smile.

"Yes," I beamed over my chow mien, satisfied. I settled back into the booth and dug in.

Back at our apartment, leftovers in the fridge, I grabbed my calendar from the desk.

"Let's set a date," I said because that was the next step.

"Do we have to set one right now?" he flinched.

"Well, yeah. Why not?" I asked, confused.

A few minutes later, with May 12, 1990 marked in my dog-eared day timer, Roger picked the phone up off the desk, turned away, and walked to the other side of the room, cord trailing behind.

"Hey, I'm en-GAGG-ed," he said to a friend, in a grim tone. He sat on the couch fiddling with a paperclip, the phone tucked between his ear and shoulder.

I pretended not to hear. My chest constricted with embarrassment. *He was probably joking*, I thought, turning my attention back to the wedding planning lists I had already started.

After he hung up, Roger grabbed my hand and slipped a twisted wire ring onto my finger. "I'll get something better as soon as I can," he said.

"It's beautiful," I laughed and kept it on, my doubts washed away by his gesture.

I got busy with the process of wedding planning, never once stopping to reflect, to wonder if we were doing the right thing. There was no one to talk sense into me, nor would I have listened. I was nothing if not completely bullheaded. My rush to get hitched and fill my baby void could not be subdued. A baby would love me as a matter of course and could not leave me. I did not ask myself if I knew how to be a good mother or if there was another way to heal. While I had rejected the religious beliefs foisted upon me as a child, the lingering shame of familial rejection was a heavy burden. I needed to be seen as an adult to my family who considered me a backslidden black sheep. I did not want to hear their criticism, but marriage might be a way to gain their acceptance. I would show them that they did not have to be ashamed of me, that Roger loved me, and wasn't just using me. They would see that I knew what I was doing. I would get married and then have a baby, in the right order.

So when I missed a period, shortly after our engagement, I did not tell anyone but Roger. I had been careless about using my diaphragm because I wasn't sure I could get pregnant again after my ectopic rupture. I was down to one working fallopian tube. In the back of my mind, I thought that if I was unable to conceive, we could adopt. Any baby would heal my heart. As it turned out, I was pregnant. Roger was excited to be a dad while I sat in stunned and shaking silence. I had done it again.

Within days, I started to spot, reddish-brown smears appeared in my underwear. I went to the urgent care clinic on a Saturday night and was sent home with strict orders to keep my feet up, but it did not help. Hours later, the spotting increased to a warm gush of blood. This baby was coming out. Roger took me back to urgent care.

"Are you two married?" the doctor asked in a conversational tone, as I lay on the exam table while his hands explored my unseen parts.

"Yes," I blurted out. Roger did not respond but looked surprised. My lie surprised me, too, and I flushed. I did not know why I lied; the doctor did not care one way or the other.

"Hmm," he said, distracted. "Ok, well, your cervix is open. It looks like you have miscarried. Have a seat here, and I'll be right back," he said, as he stripped off his gloves and walked out of the room.

Roger and I sat as instructed, holding hands, and making jokes to relieve the tension. Relief flooded my body. Now I knew I was able to get pregnant after we were married, but no one needed to know what had happened. Deep shame inflicted after my first pregnancy remained as a stain on my psyche.

In the years prior, I had started down a path of powerful independence. I abandoned religion without a backward glance. I supported myself; had started saving money, and might have parlayed my skills into a better job. Perhaps pursue an education. But I turned away from those possibilities because of my unceasing, aching loneliness, choosing to hide behind Roger and his big dreams instead of figuring out my own. The lure of being taken care of, to be behind the scenes, was seductive. Roger's ambitions were exciting and seemed like an honorable way to hide from myself; to check out. He had a creative vision, the smarts to back it up, and the will to make it happen. I did not need any of my own.

I was unable to see a future for myself alone in the world. I had no vision of who or what I could be; did not know what kinds of things there were to be. Decades later, my yoga instructor spoke to my class about achieving difficult poses; if you could picture doing a pose in your mind, she would tell us, how it would feel and how your muscles would move, then you could get there. She was right; I learned to do a backbend from standing and then rise back up by imaging how the movement would feel. Having something to reach toward, a picture in your head is vital but, at twenty-two, all I could see were babies.

But just babies, not the bills or health insurance or baggage from my own upbringing. I had no idea that it is the height of irresponsibility to have children, assuming the details will all work out. I did not realize that only ignorant, egotistical people do that, nor did I realize that I was both of those things.

So I married him. I was a misfit who would hide in the only kind of life that felt safe. I began to build a cocoon, taking the first steps to wrap up in a family of my own, ignoring the parts of myself that were neglected, because you just can't fix everything at once.

The garden wedding happened with tense family all around, in Roger's parents' yard, under a weeping willow on a luxurious expanse of green grass by a duck pond. Dad and I walked down the ribbon-lined aisle behind the pair of mallards that lived there. As we stopped at the front, he kissed my cheek and took a seat. Roger was turned away, laughing with his best man, sharing a joke. They seemed pretty hammered. I wished he was watching me with tenderness as I walked toward him. His best man gave him a nudge, and Roger turned to face me, straightening his face. We exchanged sweet vows we had written ourselves, promising to love and cherish and raise a family. My heart was full.

The officiant pronounced us man and wife.

Soon after, Roger and I headed off to The Radisson in a limousine for our wedding night. The hotel was near the Sacramento airport and provided a shuttle for our early morning flight. The place was packed when we walked in, with a long line at the desk, and a crowded lobby.

"Let's have dinner. I'm starving," I suggested as we waited for our room, sitting in a row of chairs between the hotel's front desk and bar. The smell of barbequed burgers filled my nose, contracting my empty stomach. "I never had a chance to eat today. Every single time I started to take a bite of food someone took it away from me for a picture."

"No, I don't want to," Roger refused. "I'm not hungry."

Instead of insisting, I got up and wandered over to the bar to order a Bloody Mary. At least it would have olives.

When we got our room key, I set the empty glass on the floor beside my chair and followed Roger down the hall, the cacophony of the crowded bar fading behind. We piled our suitcases in the corner. I kicked off my high heels and stripped off my dress as Roger plopped onto the king size bed with a sigh. The wedding was over; the excitement and tension of the day ebbed away in the quiet of our hotel room. We were alone at last.

As Roger relaxed, I dug into my suitcase and retrieved just the thing I had been saving for this moment, tucked it out of sight under my arm, and side-stepped into the bathroom. I unfolded the long, white nightgown received as a bridal shower gift, the silky fabric releasing in my hands. Its soft weight slunk over my body as I slipped it over my head. Delicate lace crossed my shoulders and covered my breasts, the gown swished around my legs. I gazed at my reflection in the bathroom mirror, my eyes shining with excitement. It was perfect. It was beautiful. **I** was beautiful. He would be overcome with wanting me. Our wedding night was about to be loving, sweet, and sexy. Full of unsubstantiated expectations, I crawled onto the bed where Roger was stretched out with his eyes closed and reached for him, smiling.

He pushed himself up with an elbow and swung his legs over the side of the bed. "We don't have to have sex just because it's our wedding night, do we? I have a headache," he groaned as he stood up and walked over to the television. My insides froze. He leaned over to turn on the television and, as the picture came into focus, opened the mini-bar.

"I'm hungry now. Hey, look! Let's just eat these," he exclaimed as he pulled packages of Oreos and beef jerky out of the cupboard.

"Are you kidding?" I blurted, nonplussed. I sighed, thinking about the missed burger.

"Yeah! This is fine!" he answered.

Instead of protesting, I settled back against the pillows with him, surrounded by cookie crumbs and cellophane watching something I don't remember now. Later, Roger reached for me, and we had obligatory sex I was no longer in the mood for.

During our honeymoon, Roger called his mother several times. Phoning my own never occurred to me because I thought honeymoons were supposed to be private. When I asked why he kept calling her, he said he needed to check on our cat. By the time we got home, I felt less connected to Roger than I ever had. None of the lingerie I brought along had gotten his attention. He never did hold me in his arms and tell me how happy he was to be married to me, but I believed he loved me. We moved from downtown Sacramento to a condominium closer to his parents, and I settled into a routine of commuting to work while Roger drove the other direction, to work with his dad at his home office.

Not long after the wedding, we went on a camping trip with his parents, Beth and Jerome. On this trip, I learned I would never be more important to Roger than his mother. Roger and I were wading in a beautiful, sun-dappled creek surrounded by the Sierra Nevada foothills. Huge granite boulders, warmed by the Northern California summer sun, interrupted the rushing water causing gurgles and swirls over the smooth rocks of the stream bed. Bright orange poppies and baby blue bachelor buttons dotted the surrounding fields, stretching upward, making the most of their brief stint in the sun. I climbed onto a rough, sun-warmed stone and lay back onto a flat spot to watch the day. Roger waded over with an empty picnic cup, a bottle of shampoo, and a towel.

"Want me to wash your hair?" he offered.

"Really? Yeah!" I agreed, surprised and turned on by his attentiveness. Roger did not touch me as much since the wedding and rarely with any sensuality.

I hung my head off the side of the boulder as Roger massaged the shampoo into my hair. I relaxed into his hands, as the cool creek water rinsed the heat from my scalp. The pressure of his fingers woke my body. The nearness of my in-laws kept my clothes on. With the soap bubbles vanquished and my hair wrapped in the towel, I slid off the rock and picked my way to shore, aching with desire, wondering if we could float further downstream for some privacy.

As I dried off on the bank, I heard Roger say, "Want me to do yours, too?"

"Sure!" Beth responded.

As Roger washed his mother's hair, she moaned, "Oh, Roger that feels so good."

My stomach clenched as I watched him touch her the same way he had touched me moments before, yearning doused in an instant. As it would turn out, I would always be the third wheel in their relationship.

Our sex life left me longing, just a few months into our marriage. I yearned for passion and wanted to try new things. I wanted to spend hours in bed on the weekends, playing around. I wanted to be desired. Anything I suggested to bring sensuality into our relationship was met with dismissal:

Massage book? Too weird.

Lovers' board game? Dumb.

What did he ever do with those fur-lined Velcro handcuffs? Disappeared.

I came home from a weekend away to find a Hustler magazine in his desk drawer and was furious. Not because he was looking at porn but because he did not invite me to share it. I was unable to get his attention. I was also increasingly desperate for babies. He wanted to wait, but I did not. I thought about chalking the marriage up to a mistake and moving back downtown. Embarrassment, ego, and friendship I did not want to lose; hope that it would get better kept me there. I could not bear the thought of admitting defeat and returning to a life alone.

Chapter 10
Deliverance

Several miscarriages happened before a baby stuck. My would-be babies kept falling out. Too soon after the last loss, I wasn't expecting this pregnancy to succeed, either. The doctor put me on one baby aspirin a day to balance out a possible blood chemistry cause which turned out to be the fix. Once past the first trimester danger zone, and with a strong fetal heartbeat at every check-up, I relaxed. I was having a baby. I was 25 years old when the summer of 1992 came sizzling in, with a sweating beach-ball belly in the Sacramento heat, and raging thrombose hemorrhoids. Sitz baths, *What to Expect When You're Expecting*, Lamaze classes, and anticipation beyond belief filled my days. The Lamaze teacher warned, "If you are going to the hospital and you stop and smile for the camera, you are not ready. Go back in the house. Labor is long." The snapshot taken of me beside the car shows me goofing for the camera, pretending to scream in pain, but I was ten days past due, contractions were five minutes apart, I had raw nerves bulging out of my anus, and I was going in, damn it. I carried my suitcase to the car while Roger waited in the driver's seat. I threw my bag into the back seat, and we took off. I was ready to have this baby.

Alex emerged a day later, all nine and a half pounds of him, pulled reluctantly into the light with a suction cup while I yelled my head off.

Karissa said, "He's out, you can stop yelling now. Ronna, watch. Watch him turn pink."

Panic and pain vanished as I watched the sunrise in his body while he wailed. Floodgates opened in my heart and love poured in. Alex was a self-entertainer, the calmest baby ever, after that first howling. First ones are like that, they make you think parenthood is easy so you will give them a sibling to play with. I learned early on to leave Alex alone when he was involved in a game, and he was always involved. He had more stories in his head than Roald Dahl. So we had another one. Roger wanted to wait, but I did not. I could not understand his hesitation. He knew I wanted kids and right away. That was always the plan. We were still convinced that he would sell a television show. Money would not be a problem for long. What's to worry?

Jane came along, with her big laugh, and pure joy. This kid delighted in everything. As an infant, when I held her face to face, she grabbed my ears and, with an open slobbering mouth, attempted to swallow my entire face, which earned her the nickname Beastie. And that is Jane in a nutshell. Give me life, all of it. Her big brother adored her.

One afternoon in March, about a month after Jane was born, I came home from grocery shopping, pulled into the driveway of our little duplex, and parked by the porch. Determined to carry everything in one trip, I loaded one arm up with bags and the other with Jane in her car seat and hauled the whole load inside.

"Hey, I'm home," I said to Roger as I set Jane's car seat on the floor beside Alex, where he was playing with his pile of dinosaurs, lost in his own personal *Jurassic Park*. Heading to the kitchen, fingers threaded through plastic bag handles, I spotted a handwritten envelope on my desk. I paused.

"Hi," Roger glanced up from his computer, "Oh yeah, you got a letter."

I unwound my fingers from the grocery bags and picked it up. The envelope was addressed to me in Dad's familiar scrawling hand, with no return address. My heart lurched; this must be bad news. Dad did not write letters. I ripped the envelope open and pulled the folded paper out, a photocopy of a handwritten note.

"Dear Family," it began.

"I have been HIV positive for a couple of years and was recently diagnosed with AIDS. I am starting treatment right away, but there is not much that can be done for me at this point. The doctors have given me six months to live.

Love you all,

Don/Dad"

I dropped the letter on my desk and buried my face in my hands, wailing, my body wracked with panicky sobs, more fear than tears. Profound grief hit me in the chest like a surprise whack with a baseball bat. I had spent so much time being mad at Dad and hurt and disappointed by his neglect that I had forgotten how much I loved him. Reparations had a time limit now.

"Ronna, stop it. You're going to scare the kids," Roger hissed, turning in his chair.

"Dad has AIDS," I choked.

"Oh, my God. Well, ok, I'm sorry, but don't cry in front of the kids. You're going to freak them out," he said tensely, his lips tight white around the edges.

I grabbed my keys and ran back out the front door to our postage stamp front yard.

Roger followed as far as the door, "Where are you going? What are you doing? You have to calm down, Ronna."

"I'd like to see how you'd handle it if it were your parent," I hurled back at him from the lawn, my voice quaking. I ran to the car in a panic, not knowing what to do with myself. As I slid in behind the wheel, Roger walked out onto the porch.

"Well, now we know who will be the one to walk out of this marriage first," he snapped. His words shocked me.

I couldn't cry, I couldn't not cry, and I couldn't leave.

I sat in the car in the driveway for a while. I wondered why Roger thought children shouldn't witness emotions and wondered why mine always had to be squelched. Were my feelings inappropriate? Or just the way they came out of me? I never could tell when I was being weird.

Dad's voice rang in my ears, "Get outta high gear," he would deride anytime my voice rose. "Cut the drama."

I sat in the car until familiar, numbing calm descended in my mind. I got out of the car, shut the door, and walked back into the house. Roger was back at his computer. Alex was still playing, oblivious, as his T-Rex plowed through the plant eaters. Jane was still sleeping. The groceries wouldn't put themselves away.

Susan, Karissa, and I decided to go see Dad together on Father's Day, a couple of months later. He wanted us to come. None of us wanted to go. We were dreading the trip, scared of what we were going to see. A short visit, bolstered by each other, seemed safest. There is strength in numbers.

We met at Karissa's house on the outskirts of Sacramento to fly to Los Angeles together, on June 3, 1995. I lived a few miles away from her, but

Susan had come down the night before from Portland. Roger dropped Jane and me off at Karissa's door, said good-bye and took Alex back home. We loaded our bags into the trunk of Karissa's car in the early morning light, gravel crunching under our feet. I tucked Jane's car seat and diaper bag in the back seat.

The three of us stood in the driveway by the open car doors looking at each other, faces sober and drawn, without coffee.

"Are we ready for this?" Karissa asked grimly.

"I guess," I replied, arms folded against the chill.

"It's my birthday," Susan reminded us.

We had forgotten.

"Oh God, I forgot. I am so sorry," I moaned. "Happy birthday?"

"I'm so sorry. Happy birthday, Susan," Karissa offered.

Our inadequate apologies dissipated in the air.

After an uneventful flight, we landed in L.A. and rented a car. Karissa had arranged everything beforehand. She drove us straight to Dad's condo in Glendale. None of us had visited in several years, but Karissa drove like she remembered the way, navigating the streets of L.A. at top speed. She steered the rental car down the sloped drive behind the building to the security gate, reached out, and punched his number into the keypad. The machine buzzed and a metal grid slid open to the parking garage underneath the building. Karissa whipped into a visitor parking spot, and we piled out with Jane in hand. Always the little sister, I held back assuming my sisters would take charge. Susan led the way up a white adobe staircase to the second floor. Karissa and I followed, with dread in our steps, through patches of bright sunlight and slanted shadows, past bougainvillea trailing up the wall. I cuddled Jane close, relieved to have her to hold. The front door to #214 was ajar. Susan put her hand on the doorknob and pushed it open.

"Dad?" she called softly.

"Here, come in," he responded weakly, his voice a shadow of a familiar sound.

Dad was lying on the couch, small underneath a knit throw; crusted, weeping sores on his lips. His breath caught in a sob as we walked into the living room. He began to cry and held his arms out. The most powerful force in our lives lay on the couch, unable to rise, with his arms open to us. We leaned into them, all three together; his body frail beneath the blanket. I was shaken to see him so sick, already.

We passed the day, passed the baby, searched for conversation. Susan and Karissa asked about his treatment. Dad bemoaned the rise of Newt Gingrich in Washington, D.C. Susan and Karissa exchanged a glance. Dad wasn't a Republican anymore? A couple of other visitors came and went. We took turns taking breaks and stepping outside for some air to alleviate the sadness. I overfed Jane for lack anything better to do. A guest held her upright to say hello, and she began to projectile spit-up onto the floor.

"Oops, I think she ate too much!" the visitor laughed.

I ran to clean it up, worried Dad would be angry at the mess, but he did not notice.

We were all exhausted by the time his partner, James, got home from work. We took turns saying goodbye, and I love you with hugs and kisses, cautiously avoiding Dad's sores, trying to be tender with his fragile body. Susan, Karissa, Jane, and I left to go to our hotel room by the airport. After a quick dinner at the hotel restaurant, we went to our room and collapsed into sleep. The next morning, we were up and to the airport for an early flight home, quiet over coffee, lost in our thoughts, and anxious to go. There did not seem to be much to say.

Standing on the curb at the Sacramento airport, waiting for Karissa's husband, Gary, to pick us up, Susan blurted, "I just can't believe this. I can't believe he did this," shaking her head in frustration.

"Susan, people don't decide to be gay. Some people are just gay," I snapped, instantly exasperated at the religious blame insinuated in her statement. I had no patience for the argument I assumed was coming: homosexuality is a sin, a bad choice, this situation was Dad's own fault.

"I don't entirely disagree with you…" she began but said nothing more as I turned away, unwilling to hear her out. I did not even give her a chance to explain.

We went our separate ways, relieved the trip was over.

Dad's health bounced back a little bit over the summer, thanks to infusion therapy. He was well enough to visit his parents in Bend, Oregon one last time, where he bought a burial plot next to theirs. James was by his side day and night, except for Dad's visit to Bend. He wasn't welcome there, even though he was Dad's partner and his caretaker. James took care of Dad for months, cleaned up the vomit and the shit, coordinated his medical care, went to every doctor's appointment, and called 911, occasionally, when nothing else could be done. And still, there was no room in my grandparents' heart or home for him.

James called in November. "Don is in the hospital again. He won't be coming home this time. You should come," he said.

Susan and Karissa and I took another early morning flight to L.A., this time going straight to the hospital. I left Jane at home, unwilling to navigate an AIDS ward with an eight-month-old. We arranged ourselves around Dad's room, terrified to touch any surface, uncertain what to say. Nurses hurried in and out. Very sick men attached to IVs wandered the hall, stopping to peer in the doorway, seeming unsure where they were. Dad was distracted but coherent; any conversation was difficult amidst all the activity. I leaned against the side rail of his bed to hear him and realized there was dried blood under my arm. A moment of panic flooded my body. I did not want to freak out, but inside I was freaking out. Could you get AIDS from touching dried blood with your forearm?

"Um, there's some, um, blood here," I gestured to the nurse.

She bustled over, larger than life.

"Its fine, its fine. Don't worry," the nurse reassured in a sing-song voice as she wiped down the rail. She seemed accustomed to scared people.

Overwhelmed with fear and anxiety, faced with the heartbreaking devastation of AIDS all around, the three of us needed to breathe. We stepped out to get some lunch in the hospital café. There was no escaping Dad's reality at this point. There was no outcome for him other than death, and soon. Susan and Karissa were staying overnight to be there when our grandparents flew in the next day, but I was flying home that night. Jane was still nursing, and I did not have a pump; my breasts got fuller as the afternoon wore on. After lunch, Susan and Karissa went to their hotel room to rest, and I went back to see Dad by myself, before going to the airport.

I pulled a chair up beside his bed; knowing it was the last time I would ever see him alive. The ward was quieter now, the nurses elsewhere. We chatted about this and that, about Alex and Jane, the new carpet in his condo. James was on his way to pick me up, our time together was almost over. Words needed to be said. I needed to hear that he loved me, that he saw me, and knew we would never see each other again. I needed to know I mattered to him.

I attempted to turn the conversation to a more personal place, wanting to say I'm so sad you are dying, you were always my hero; hoping for warmth in return, wanting to tell him how much I loved him.

I awkwardly choked out, "You mean so much to me."

The words died in my throat as he turned away and clicked on the television with the remote. I was stunned, unable to speak as he began to watch the news.

James arrived. "Ready to go?" he asked.

"Yes," I whispered.

"Take Ronna by the condo so she can see the new carpet on your way to the airport. It's seafoam green," Dad said. "Love you. Bye."

"Love you, Dad. Bye," I said and followed James out to the car.

"Do you want to go by the condo?" James asked gently, as he pulled onto the freeway.

"No," I replied, staring out the window at dirt colored L.A. whipping by. "Please just take me to the airport."

As the plane spanned California, my lactating breasts bulged and leaked; the pressure of overly full glands intensely painful. I leaned my head back and closed my eyes, tears, and milk flowing. The passenger next to me adjusted her seatbelt, bumping my arm which jostled my breast, and I gasped in pain.

"Oh, I'm sorry, did I hurt you?" she asked, concerned.

"It's ok," I said. "I just need to get home."

I explained my day, my dad, and my screaming boobs.

"I'll never see him again," I admitted.

When I got home, Jane turned her head away from my breast. She wasn't hungry. I milked myself, squirting hot streams into a towel until the pressure was relieved, hands dripping, and the towel soaked.

Three weeks later, on December 12th, 1995, the phone rang at 2:00 in the morning. I lay in bed feigning sleep, listening to the ring coming from the living room, knowing it was James. I did not get up to answer. The phone rang again at 6:00 am, and this time I got up. Dad had died in hospice, in James's arms, while he sang him to sleep. Dad was out of pain. Shadows lifted. It was over.

Dad's funeral was on a bone-chilling, wind-blasted April day in Bend. As I stood next to James on the cemetery lawn, squinting into the whipping wind, he said with a smirk, "Brrrr, Don would have hated this wind."

"He sure would," I laughed.

Someone had decided that Susan, Karissa, and I should each speak at the funeral. A few weeks before, Karissa called me.

"Do you, ummm, need help with what to say at the funeral?" she asked hesitantly. "Susan and I can help you if you want."

Maybe they thought I was going to say something crazy since I no longer pretended to be a Christian. Maybe they thought I would go on a pro-gay rant, which I had to admit was a possibility. I did not know or ask for the reason behind the offer.

"No, thank you. I don't need any help," I snipped, annoyed.

"Okay... well, let us know if you do," she offered again, sounding worried.

"Yeah, okay," I said, as I hung up the phone.

I had a poem picked out. It seemed to me that Dad had risked everything to be himself. His choices cost him his life, but I admired him for starting over. When it was my turn to speak, I stepped to the front of the gathering, gripping my fluttering paper. I glanced at the crowd, saw my grandmother's stricken face and began:

To laugh is to risk appearing the fool
To weep is to risk appearing sentimental
To reach for another is to risk involvement
To expose your ideas, your dreams
Before a crowd is to risk their loss
To love is to risk not being loved in return
To live is to risk dying
To believe is to risk despair
To try is to risk failure

But risks must be taken because the
Greatest hazard in life is to risk nothing
The people who risk nothing, do nothing
Have nothing, are nothing
They may avoid suffering and sorrow
But they cannot learn, feel, change
Grow, love, live
Chained by their attitudes, they are slaves
They have forfeited their freedom
Only a person who risks is free
-by William Arthur Ward (attributed to)

After Dad's death, I began to have sporadic, soul-quaking nightmares about him that left me terrified. The dreams were traumatic, disturbing, but most were vague and unformed. Early one morning, I startled awake, yanked to reality; sweating and shaking, my heart pounding, and my stomach sick. The sound of scathing derision in Dad's voice still echoed in my head. He had been raking me over the coals for some misstep. Accusations hurled, no chance given to respond or defend, helpless in the bulls-eye of his scorn; chest so tight breath cannot escape, words cannot form, body and mind locked in a vise of paralyzing numbness, an internal icebox hiding my wrecked, wounded, angry soul. *Not fair, not fair, not fair, not fair. Love me. Why don't you love me?* Nowhere to go but inside.

"What's wrong?" Roger asked, from where he stood at the bathroom sink.

"Another dream about Dad," I said, gasping for air.

"Ugh, I'm sorry," he responded around a mouthful of toothpaste.

I got up to get a cup of coffee. Roger was always up first and started the pot every morning.

Sporadic dreams continued for a few months. They increased in intensity until one night, something shifted. The scene began as usual. Dad started to criticize and accuse.

I stood up.

I faced him.

My heart pounded out of my chest, my voice quivered, my gut quaked, and my knees buckled. I couldn't speak, and I couldn't not speak.

"You-you-you can't treat me this way. You c-c-c-can't talk to me like that. Go away and don't come back."

As these simple childlike stammers left my mouth, Dad vanished like smoke.

The dreamed fear in my body was as real as it would have been, had I ever confronted him alive. As the dream faded, fear left. A wave of relief carried me to peaceful wakefulness.

I never dreamed about him again.

Chapter 11
Fantasy Life

Life with two tiny kids and another one on the way, due to a poorly timed hormone surge and missed birth control pill, consumed me. Diapers and walks to the park, preschool, and playdates. Stacks of storybooks, *Sesame Street*, piles of plastic dinosaurs, and camping trips filled our days. No project was too messy, no puddle off limits, no story time too long. The salty tang of fresh, homemade playdough wafted up from the warm plop as I sank my hands in, kneading it together with watercolor paint. I loved to play at least as much as Alex and Jane did.

Jane begged for a Barbie when she turned three. I was not excited about the toy, but let her spend her birthday money on one because I remembered all too well how it felt to yearn for the forbidden. Jane bee-lined to the backyard with her new doll. I followed and watched as she took scissors to the blonde plastic hair and a gloppy blue paintbrush to its face, the minuscule pink mini dress lost in the dirt.

"Look, Mommy, NOW she's beautiful," Jane said, dreamily, swishing Barbie's bald head around in the fish pond.

"What's her name?" I questioned.

"Shallow," Jane answered, and I relaxed about any adverse effects of Barbie's unrealistic beauty standards.

We set up a trampoline in the backyard, a perfect platform for games of all kinds. I sat in the middle of the bouncy black surface as Alex and Jane rolled and jumped around me. Jane's favorite spot was in my lap, in the middle of the trampoline, while Alex hopped around us in his swishy, pink polyester nightgown. To my great amusement, he enjoyed wearing it with no underwear on, because it felt good. Our house became a free for all play center. I watched and learned as my children swirled around me. They played with abandon, and I relished every moment.

In those early years of parenting, the writings of Tom Robbins and Joseph Campbell gave me mind-expanding philosophy and humor. Educators Alfie Kohn and Bev Bos and author Alice Miller provided an understanding of child development. My brain and emotions found new places to live in their words. Ideas I had always felt to be right found structure and substance. I absorbed the newfound information and broader perspectives of the world with keen interest. There was no developmental stage for instilling the fear of Hell. Children did not have to be punished. Sex education could be devoid of guilt and shame. I was shocked to learn while reading Joseph Campbell's *The Power of Myth*, that many of the Bible stories I had been taught as a child were common themes throughout religions all over the world. While I had already abandoned the precepts of religion, exposure to a broader picture of cultural and historical beliefs left me bitter at the constrictions and fabricated fears of my own childhood. My determination to protect my own children from the mores of religion grew. They would know nothing about it.

While I was immersed with our children, Roger was occupied in his office, a room attached to the garage. Ants crawled in a train across the length of his office wall and out the back, as he sat staring at his computer screen. He retired to the living room couch about 5:00 every afternoon, exhausted as if from digging ditches.

"What is going on?" I worried as he lay on the couch again. Alex and Jane were playing *Lion King* on their bunk beds in the next room.

"What do you mean?" he questioned.

"You seem so unhappy," I hesitated. My concern and frustration at Roger's apparent depression was increasing. The happier I got, the more detached he became.

"I'm not unhappy. What are you talking about?" Roger retorted testily.

"Happy people don't lay down on the couch, exhausted at 5:00 in the afternoon after having done nothing all day. And you have gotten so heavy, I'm worried about your health," I expressed, skirting around how appalled I was at his weight gain.

His recent media project had not produced the results he had hoped for. He had turned down an offer from a production company in Hollywood because it wasn't enough money. I couldn't help. Roger couldn't watch the kids and work at the same time if I were to get a job and, anyway, I was weeks away from giving birth to baby number three. If he got a job, he would not have time to pursue his own projects, which was the path to his professional success and our life of financial security. The best option seemed to be to hold onto hope that Roger would sell an idea. I had no doubts about his talent. Even though I was a firm non-believer, I began to live by faith once again. I had unwittingly switched allegiances from faith in an invisible God to my husband's promises. Turning off the little voice in my head that told me to make a plan, I buckled myself into the back seat of my own life.

While waiting for Hollywood to make a better offer, Roger worked with his father creating educational science media. Jerome was a brilliant biologist and a quietly powerful man. Smart, sarcastic, and controlled, he was single-minded about his work. With his fly-away comb-over and wire-rimmed glasses sliding down his nose, he spent countless hours growing organisms in leaky aquariums on his back deck. Jerome had invented a system for filming microscopic life in real time; a complex system of cameras attached to microscopes attached to tanks swarming with green and brown life. The resulting footage showed a surreal realm, invisible to the naked eye, where undulating, transparent creatures propelled themselves through the murk. Jerome showed me the world through his microscopes, and I was enthralled; as was he, to watch me learn.

His films needed to keep up with technology to continue selling, and that is where Roger fit in. Roger taught himself how to do computer animation to advance their media products. He was that smart. Filmstrips evolved to video, then to CDs, and online streaming. Roger seemed miserable working with his father, or maybe he was miserable being married to me. He seemed frustrated and hopeless. So he ate. And ate. Hand to mouth, over and over. I couldn't figure out what the problem was, exactly.

August in Roseville hit the 110-degree mark again, as we sat on wobbly, white plastic lawn chairs under the giant sycamore in our backyard, sipping drinks with Ed, a preschool dad, who had brought his kids over to play. My swollen breasts lolled on top of my pregnant belly, which spread over my lap. Rivulets of sweat soaked into my bra and underwear.

"Ah God, it's hot," Ed moaned, tilting his beer bottle to his mustachioed mouth.

"Ugh, terrible," Roger agreed, rubbing his bare feet in the dirt. "Mom offered to buy us a swamp cooler for the house, but I said no. Setting those things up is a pain in the ass," he laughed.

My breath caught in my throat. He had turned down a free air conditioner for no reason other than he couldn't be bothered to install it, while I sweltered under the weight of his third burgeoning baby? I couldn't believe it.

"You asshole," I hissed.

Roger froze and stared at me as if seeing my condition for the first time. Ed smirked and looked away. I felt my response come out of me by itself. I rehearsed every conversation with Roger in my head if I thought I might offend or upset him, so my expletive surprised us both. The swamp cooler was set up in a matter of days.

A couple of months later, with contractions coming regularly, Alex and Jane went to their grandparents' house, and the midwives came to ours. I had hired midwives specializing in home birth because individual health insurance had become prohibitively expensive in California and we could no longer afford it. We lived seconds away from the fire station and minutes from the nearest emergency room, so I figured if the unthinkable happened help would be within reach since health insurance was not.

My water broke about 11:00 pm and sweet Marie appeared just after midnight, an All Saints baby instead of Halloween. Sleeping in my own bed and using my own bathroom after giving birth was amazing. After the delivery was over, the top layer of bedding and waterproof sheet were peeled off. Clean, dry bedding awaited beneath. I rolled over and went to sleep.

Marie was beautiful, with round pink cheeks and a rosebud mouth. Calm and precious, there was something about her that captured a place in my heart I did not know was there. She could sleep with her siblings howling around her and the vacuum running under her swing. Alex and Jane took turns holding her on the couch, but she was Jane's baby. Jane held her with fascination, patience, love, and complete ownership.

As the children grew, I found many ways to distract myself, but there were a few times when I admitted the deep unhappiness beneath the surface. Roger always had to be the center of attention at his parents' house for family get-togethers, which left me singlehandedly juggling tiny children while he performed. After one such event, I took a deep breath and summoned my courage on the way home. Any semblance of conflict made it difficult for me to get words to come out of my mouth.

"I really need your help at these family dinners," I broached, my heart quivering as I anticipated his defensive response. "You just ignore the kids and me, and I end up taking care of everyone by myself. You don't help me at all."

"Oh, I just forget about you," he admitted.

I looked out the window, surprised at the bald truth of his dismissal. Despair settled heavily in my chest as the blur of dry, white parched Sacramento Valley roadside weeds passed by.

"Well, I don't want to have any more kids unless that changes," I stated bluntly. We had always planned on having four.

"I'll help more. I will," Roger promised.

At that moment, I knew I should have my tubes tied, go back to school as soon as it was feasible, and set myself up to take care of our children with or without him. My inner realist told me to take charge now. But taking those steps would tell Roger that I did not believe in his ability to succeed. I did not want to hurt his feelings. I would also be admitting to myself that I had lost faith in him, that I was planning life without him, plotting an escape, and a new life as a divorced, single mom. I would never be willing to support him while he dreamed. I knew this. The result would be me working full time and struggling, while he would likely live at his parents' house with our children. They would take care of him, and I would be forgotten and alone.

I could not face that eventuality. I wanted to believe that Roger would come through, that the fantasy we were spinning was real. I gambled that Roger would be a successful television producer and make us rich, so I could stay home and play with the kids. Believing was easier than change.

When Marie was a year old, we moved to Bellingham, Washington to get away from the heat and increasing congestion of the Sacramento Valley, and from Roger's parents, who had grown more and more distant as our family grew. They were not particularly interested in being grandparents, so there was no reason to stay close. They made it clear that they were not available for babysitting after Jane was born and three was out of the question. Their aloofness was less insulting from farther away. Roger and I were excited about the move. He did not express any concern about being so far away from his parents, although his mother acted like it wasn't happening until the U-Haul was loaded.

Moving day came. Roger and I headed north on Interstate 5, leaving Roseville, California for our new home in Bellingham, Washington, our teal minivan loaded with babies, suitcases and diapers. Roger's friend, Peter, followed in the U-Haul with everything else we owned, including the cats. We caravanned along in the slow lane, trying to keep the vehicles together through bumper to bumper Portland traffic. The kids were buckled into their car seats surrounded by juice boxes and capless markers, while Roger groaned in the passenger seat. Somehow he had gotten food poisoning.

As I maneuvered through the hurtling stream of vehicles, Roger yelled, "PULL OVER, PULL OVER, PULL OVER!"

"Oh my God, ok, ok!" I responded in a panic, turned on my blinker and swerved to the shoulder in one motion. Tires skidded in the gravel as I white-knuckled to a halt. Roger flung open his door and barreled out, ran a few steps into the weeds, and began to heave, as the U-Haul sped past. I sighed. We would never catch up with Peter and the U-Haul. He had no idea what exit to take to my mother's house, where we were supposed to stop for dinner. *How had Roger gotten so sick? Was it the chicken he ate last night?* I was still gripping the steering wheel.

"What's going on, Mommy?" Alex asked, as he and his little sisters, Jane and Marie, strained against their car seat straps to watch their father vomit into the dry, end-of-summer weeds by the side of the road.

"Daddy doesn't feel good," I reassured in a calm mommy voice, while sweat blossomed and spread in my armpits. The steering wheel gamely resisted my attempts to bend it in half.

Roger lurched back to the van and crawled in, slumped in his seat, and shuddered, deathly pale.

"You ok?" I asked with concern. *God, he was really sick. Fuck.*

He nodded, his eyes closed.

"Ready?" I asked again, not wanting to leave if he had another wave coming up.

"Yes, just go," he snapped.

I turned on the blinker, tensely watching for an opening in the eighty miles per hour traffic. I hesitated, terrified. Merging into this screaming, rush hour stream seemed impossible. Our minivan did not accelerate quickly, especially when I was driving, and my babies were in here. My pulse accelerated as I waited for an opening in the onslaught of speeding cars, my upper lip beaded with sweat, my foot hovered over the gas pedal.

"Just go! What are you waiting for?" Roger burst out aggressively. "I would have had us back on the road by now-"

"Hey! SHUT UP!" I bellowed at full volume, my voice projecting through the van.

Fury at the additional pressure calmed my nerves instantly. Tense silence descended as I merged smoothly into traffic. The kids had never heard me yell at Roger before. I guess I had to experience a life-threatening situation to do it. As soon as we were back on the road, I calmed down and reverted to my tamped down self, to keep the peace, and continue weaving the fantasy of our marriage. Keeping the part of myself that had any gumption under wraps seemed like the safest course of action because to insist on change means having to do it yourself.

We settled into a big barn of a house on Sehome Hill with an apple tree in the yard. The sun rose behind Mt. Baker every morning and sunsets reflected off its snowy peak in the evening. Deer wandered through our yard; the Pacific Northwest air was clean and crisp. There was no traffic. I thought we would fit right in with the hippie crowd, but we were way too square, and my social ineptness had followed me. My fear of public school prompted me to put the kids into an alternative school which did not seem to have any actual curriculum. After a couple of years of trying to make it work, I gave up. With Alex behind socially and Jane behind academically, I quelled my fears and put them into public school.

Birth control and health insurance had failed me again. Another homebirth, one hour start to finish, Oliver weighed in at ten pounds and seven ounces, and it was time to stop having babies. They kept getting bigger. We were living hand to mouth, still. Roger always had a new script idea, none of which ever panned out. By this time, I was terrified about our future. He continued to work with Jerome, for which he was paid quarterly royalties. Since his pay was based on media sales, the amount fluctuated. I paid our bills in advance, three months at a time, and whatever was left was what we lived on. I had managed our finances this way for years, but the situation was becoming untenable.

What began as a cocoon, a safe haven, had become a prison. The babies I had surrounded myself with left me unable to do anything other than care for them. Working outside the home was impossible, even though Roger was always there. He did not clean or keep track of the children; couldn't remember to put hot things out of reach of toddlers. He did not want to teach the kids to ride a bike or swim, all the stuff he grew up doing. He lost children more than once. One day when Oliver was two, Roger left him unbuckled in the stroller and wandered off in the middle of Target. I had the store in lockdown before I found Oliver playing around in the racks. I even had someone call me from a park one time, threatening to call the police because my toddlers were alone on the playground. Roger had wandered off to the other side of the park, across a parking lot to watch Alex's soccer practice, and left them alone. By a lake. I screamed at him through the phone, sobbing in panic and disbelief.

I was trapped. I couldn't see a way out of the dismal situation I had created. Day after day, I resigned myself to having faith that Roger would sell a project as I watched the kids clamber into his lap for his ever-ready hugs and kisses and I love yous, the type of affection he never received from his own father. His eagerness to patiently explain intricate plot points to every movie they watched together lit their imaginations on fire and jumpstarted their intellects. He carved the pumpkins, cut the Christmas trees, and cooked delectable dinners. They adored their father. I could not dismantle our family. So I kept hoping. I did not know what else to do.

When the kids weren't around, my attempts at discussion about budgets or a stable income were shut down right along with any conversation about our obligatory, half-hearted sex life. I hated the feeling of physical disconnectedness. My helplessness and hopelessness remained as my fear and anger grew.

Like many unhappy marriages, we were companionable in a lot of ways. I loved the way the kids spread out through the house and yard, creating play spaces and private spots, making up games and torturing each other out of earshot of me. Up at dawn every day, Roger bounced out of bed and cheerfully bounded downstairs to make breakfast. We had little physical connection, but I tried to pretend it was because we were so busy with kids. A friend offered to babysit for the weekend so Roger and I could spend a night in Seattle, and I took her up on it, excited at the prospect. We never went anywhere alone.

We wandered around Pike Street Market, inching our way through the crowds with waxed paper bags of hot doughnuts. I weaved through a group of tourists and Roger called, "Wait for me! I can't get through as the crowd as fast as you can." He had a panicked look in his eyes, his face a ghostly pale. "I need to find a bathroom," he whispered when he caught up with me.

He always got nervous away from home. I did not know why he was so uncomfortable. I was confused by it and frustrated, as well. We were supposed to be having fun. We followed the restroom sign down the stairs and then continued strolling along the waterfront where the crowds were thinner. I remembered to slow down while we explored the shops together.

Later, I got dressed up in black leather pants, a black sleeveless tunic with leather trim, and black stilettos. Lipstick, even. I took him to the Buenos Aires Grill for Argentine steak and tango watching, ready for date night. We got through dinner. The food was out of this world, and the dancers were smooth as hot silk. I glanced away from the show to see Roger watching me with a pained look in his eyes.

"Thank you for dressing up for me. I appreciate it. I know you did all this for me, but I just can't," he almost whispered.

I felt the painful burn of humiliation spread through my chest, feeling foolish in my leather and lipstick. We went back to the Warwick Hotel, a small, retro-glam place with spectacular views of the Space Needle. Roger turned on the television to watch a science fiction movie he had seen a million times before. I lay on the cushy bed, staring out the window at the Space Needle, desperately sad, wondering if he would ever want me. *But*, I thought, *to be fair, he doesn't feel well.* I tried to convince myself it was nothing more than that.

Two days before Oliver turned five years old, Jerome fell off the roof of their house while working on the gutters and suffered a head injury. We were uncertain how severe the injury was and waited to hear from Roger's mother with instructions to come or not. Roger and I lay awake, waiting in the night. The phone rang.

"You better come," she said.

Jerome's fall had severed his brain from the stem. There was no hope of survival. Roger pulled on his jeans and grabbed the duffel bag he had already packed. He went into his office and clicked purchase on the flight leaving at dawn and drove through the night to the Seattle airport. He rented a car upon arrival in Sacramento and drove straight to the hospital where his family waited. Roger got there in time to say goodbye, and the doctors turned off the respirator. Roger held Jerome's hand and talked to him as he took his last breath.

Nothing was ever the same after that. Jerome was gone, and we were all heartbroken. The kids had lost their grandfather, and our family had lost its rudder. Days later, I sat in my car during Jane's soccer practice, soaking up the heat of the afternoon sun through the window, savoring a few moments alone. Roger called from home. I told him I had a dream the night before about Jerome and his loss hit me. I began to cry.

'What is wrong?" Roger yelled. "Why are you having a breakdown? I'm fine."

I caught my breath at his sudden attack, my tears dissolving. I loved Jerome, too. He was the father I did not have. His willingness to provide Roger with work that supported our family was a stabilizing force in our lives. I knew we would be up a creek without his guidance, a burgeoning fear that was secondary to the deep missing of him that was already settling into my heart like a cavern. I was not fine. And I knew better, Roger wasn't fine, either.

Roger took over management of their business, a difficult task without Jerome. Then the economy tanked. I had no idea how bad things were financially. I wasn't in that loop.

His mother, Beth, visited us in Bellingham. She and Roger and I sat at the dining room table, discussing the future of their business, which looked grim. Beth mentioned the $43,000 Roger had borrowed over the last year, and how that would be reimbursed.

"Wait, what?" I stopped the conversation, turning to Roger. "You borrowed $43,000 *without telling me*?"

He looked at his mother. She looked at me and nodded. "Yes." She answered even though I was talking to Roger. I do not know if she realized

Roger had kept this from me, but he sat silently as she responded.

"*I want a divorce. From both of you*," is what I wanted to say. But instead, I sat in stunned silence. They both stared back at me, waiting for me to leave, the three of us at the empty dining room table. Roger and Beth resumed talking to each other, and I retreated, dismissed, wondering how much longer I could stay married.

Chapter 12
No Safe Place

About that time, Mom got sick. Susan, Karissa, and I had taken her shopping for a new birthday outfit, as was our tradition. She picked out a denim duster with an embroidered waistband. She struggled with the closure around her waist, which was surprising as she had always been slim.

"Mid-life expansion, I guess," she shrugged, looking kind of pissed off about it.

Soon after, however, she noticed that even her skin did not fit anymore. The usual padding of fat between skin and bone had vanished; her flesh hung empty, despite the thickness around her waist. She struggled to eat more than a mouthful, feeling full after a few bites. A doctor's appointment was made. Susan called me with the stunning results. An enormous malignant sarcoma had infiltrated Mom's abdomen. Fully tentacled into her blood supply, the tumor was stealing her nutrients. Starving her. We were all in shock that such a thing could grow without her knowledge. She felt fine.

Surgical oncologist, Dr. Kent Williamson of OHSU in Portland, Oregon, was Mom's surgeon. Dr. Williamson inspired confidence; no other doctor in the area performed this type of surgery. He had reviewed her scans over and over, consulted with a team of doctors, and plotted every step of the multi-faceted procedure. He was as prepared as possible to detach Mom's alien guest. The whole family was anxious and worried, but Mom was calm. She knew she was in good hands and her faith allowed her to accept whatever outcome was to be. She refused to worry. Whatever happened would be God's will.

The first step of the operation was a venal reroute, performed by the first medical team. They would detach and reattach the main artery that fed the sarcoma, so that Mom's blood supply would bypass the tumor, cutting off its source of nutrient. Then Dr. Williamson and his team would begin the painstaking disconnection of every minuscule vein feeding the sarcoma, lasering the connecting capillaries as they simultaneously eased this monstrosity out of Mom's abdomen. Great care had to be taken not to disrupt the sarcoma in any way so every cancer cell could be removed.

The morning of her surgery, Susan, Karissa, and I took Mom to the hospital very, very early, up the hill to OHSU. (Whoever decided to build a hospital at the top of a straight uphill? That hill looked like something out of *Hop on Pop*.) Susan and Mom got out at the entrance while Karissa and I parked the car. We were all in good spirits. Hopeful. Mom was whisked away to pre-op as I sat with my sisters in the private waiting area.

A nurse in green scrubs and hat poked his head out of the pre-op room, "Ok, you can come in and wish her well now."

We marched in, ready with hugs and kisses and positivity. Mom sat on the side of the bed, hunched over, tubes already inserted in her back.

"Hi, Mama," I said, touching her hand. "You ok?"

She moaned. Quiet settled over her. She was silent.

"I love you, Mama," I reassured. "We'll see you soon."

She did not respond. We filed back out for one final discussion with the anesthesiologist.

"Can we watch?" Karissa asked. "Is there an observatory?"

"You don't want to watch this," he shook his head.

"I do," I responded, thinking the surgery would be fascinating to see. I was not squeamish.

The doctor shook his head again, aghast at our naiveté, "Absolutely not."

Mom would be in surgery for hours; we went back up to the main waiting room to sit. And sit. The gift shop, the cafeteria, walk the halls, no way to read a book. Neither my brain nor my body could settle down. The phone in the nurses' station rang every hour or two with a report. So far, so good. The cousins came by. As we sat to chat with them, the phone rang again. There was a problem. Dr. Williamson would come out to speak with us as soon as he could. Cousins and sisters sat back down on the orange vinyl. Quiet now. Tense.

Dr. Williamson appeared shortly. He sat in the armchair facing us and explained, "Rae's blood loss got ahead of us and her heart rate flat-lined. One of our cardiologists was in the unit and was able to resuscitate her, but she was out for about fifteen minutes."

Dr. Williamson paused and turned his head away, hand to mouth. I noticed his lips quivering. And his scrubs were clean. He must have changed.

He turned back to us and continued, "At that point, we had to just carve the sarcoma out to remove it as quickly as possible. We stopped the bleeding as much as we could. She's in ICU now. The next few hours are crucial."

I sat stunned. Reading between the lines, while Mom's body cavity was wide open, her heart stopped. A cardiologist, who happened to be walking by, got on top of the table, on top of her, and pumped Mom's heart by hand until it started back up. Then the surgical team hacked the ten-pound sarcoma out of her body, packed her abdomen full of gauze, stitched her up, and sent her to ICU to live or die. Her blood loss was extreme. Even if she pulled through, the end results were unknown. Mom had been without oxygen for fifteen minutes; she could have suffered brain damage, the worst case scenario to my mind. Worse than death. I could not imagine my tough, stoic, unflappable mother as anything but alive and well. Losing her might be easier.

Susan, Karissa, and I were invited to go down to ICU. Silently in the elevator, leaning against the walls, we descended and walked through the bunker-like cement hallway, following curt arrows. We reached a set of heavy glass doors. A voice came through an intercom, "Who are you?"

We gave our names and said, "Here to see Rae Fisher."

The doors buzzed open, and we entered. The first room to the right was a frenzy of activity. Three nurses surrounded a bed, a bed that held the body of my mother. Each of the nurses was doing several things at once, sweat poured down their faces as they yelled instructions to each other across the room. They did not notice when we entered. Behind the bed was a bank of monitors, beeping and flashing. We stood still, the three of us, in the doorway.

"We are not supposed to be in here," I thought to myself. "What were they thinking, sending us down here? Someone made a mistake."

Then I realized.

We had been allowed in to say good-bye. Karissa, Susan and I huddled together by the door, watching the heroes in scrubs. Mom, what looked like it could be, might be, my Mom, lay still, encompassed by tubes and tape and gauze and sheet. We couldn't get anywhere near her. We watched the nurses trying desperately to save her life. There was no room for us. After a while we went back up to the waiting room, rattled. The cousins left, and we spread out on the benches in the deserted hospital hallway to wait out the night. The hours ticked.

We dozed on the hallway benches. Each of us, at different times, wandering down to sit with Mom. I perched on a stool by her side, taking in the blipping, blinking screens, mysterious tubes running under her sheet and under her skin, and the ventilator tube sagging the corner of her pale mouth. There was no safe place to touch her.

"It's ok, Mama, if you want to go," I whispered, tears in my throat. "You don't have to come back if you don't want to. I love you."

I felt sure that she heard me.

I wouldn't want to come back to this, I thought as I looked around at the blinking monitors. *This is too hard.*

Early in the morning, Dr. Williamson stopped by our camp. "She's as stable as she can be for now," he said. "Go home." He looked us up and down. "And take showers," he added with a smile.

We did. We went to Mom's house, took showers and naps and returned to the hospital, refreshed and ready to face whatever was going to happen next. Mom's incision had to be reopened to unpack the mountain of gauze left inside and to staunch any bleeding. She went back into surgery without having been brought to consciousness. A day or so later, her vital signs were stable, and she was moved to a rehabilitation unit of the hospital for a month long stay she wouldn't remember.

Mom's digestive system had been shoved aside by the sarcoma for so long that it took a while to resettle back into a normal configuration. Her tubes rebelled against any input, hurtling liquids and medications out without warning in all directions. She was still hooked up to more machines and monitors than I could track; tubes, IVs and stents everywhere. I went home and came back. I learned to change bedsheets with her inert body still in them. I wiped and cleaned and stroked her hair. I stood up to an abusive nurse and had her taken off duty. I was there.

Mom stabilized. I drove north toward home, exhausted, relieved, and grateful to have been there for her, glad to have rallied around her with my sisters. As my minivan sped through the green countryside of Southern Washington State, I reflected on the emotional roller-coaster of the previous weeks. The irony was not lost on me that when a person's insides explode through no fault of their own, it is okay to show them love. Their wounds are accepted as an unfortunate trauma. My own life-threatening pregnancy had been the result of sexual misconduct; therefore it was my own fault, my sin, and thus I had not qualified. I cared for my mother the way I needed her to care for me. Decades later, I could be who she could not. Isn't it interesting the way we end up being who we needed?

Chapter 13
Closets

After my fourth child, Oliver was born, the baby weight wasn't dropping off as it had in the past. I loved my little family and knew the extra pounds shouldn't matter but felt as though my body was letting me down. I remembered Dad saying that if you were fat, you had no one to blame but yourself. I remember him telling me that he would leave Mom if she ever gained weight. My heaviness as a teenager had concerned her greatly. Not my depression or withdrawal, just my extra pounds. Being fat wasn't okay, and I had always been the only fat one in the family.

I wanted to not worry about the baby weight, but decades of emotional starvation and belief that I was unlovable if I was not thin had taken their toll on my mental health. Self-acceptance wasn't an option.

Nothing had snapped back into place down below, either; my vaginal walls were weak and stretched, and I began to feel panicked. I attacked the problem of my body full force, intent on fixing it. Up before dawn every day to run the trails of Sehome Hill Arboretum and then fend off hunger with coffee until time for egg whites and veggies at 10:00 am. A gallon of water and a big salad dressed with plain vinegar at 2:00 pm, then Ashtanga yoga at 5:00 pm; no dinner.

After a few months of this regimen, my extra weight was gone, and my vagina was like new. Nineteen percent body fat, the Bod Pod scanner said; the body fat percentage of an athlete. I contorted myself in front of the mirror, searching for cellulite wobbles and fat bulges. They were gone. I weighed myself every morning and every evening, for good measure. Everything was high and tight, if you know what I mean, except for my sagging stomach skin, which hung in wrinkled folds from above my navel. I felt fantastic other than the nagging hunger, but I still couldn't get Roger's attention. Somewhere in the back of my mind, I thought if I could just be perfect maybe he would want me. Or maybe I would want me. But I had achieved the best version of my physical self, and it still wasn't enough. He did not care. Soccer dads had started sidling up to me during games, making conversation. They almost always ended up complaining about their wives' weight. I wondered why they were telling me.

One evening, while the kids were setting the table for dinner, nine-year-old Alex asked, "Should I get a plate for you, Mom?" His words hit me like a punch in my empty gut. *Had I skipped that many dinners?* I thought. *Holy shit.*

I had stopped eating dinner with my family, the holy grail of togetherness. My children were becoming accustomed to having one of those mothers who doesn't eat. I knew women like that; my mother-in-law was one of them. They never relaxed around food, counting every calorie with grim determination, and make no mistake, they were counting yours, too. Constant vigilance was required to remain fat-free. I did not want to be one of those women and I sure as hell did not want to be that kind of mother. My daughters deserved a better example. So did my sons. *Fuck this*, I thought. *What was I trying to prove?* I made an instant decision.

"Yes, Alex, set a place for me," I replied without hesitation. I never skipped dinner again.

Being a size 0 had gotten me nowhere but paranoid. My weight bounced up right away, of course. When I twisted my hips in front of the mirror or stretched my leg onto the counter to check the size of my thigh and buttock fat blobs, I could see they were creeping back. Not wanting to watch, I quit looking. I also stopped getting on the scale and going to yoga every day. Hitting the gym a few times a week would have to be good enough. There had to be a reasonable way to feel good in my skin without making myself insane by constantly starving and monitoring my ass dimples.

Clothes were the answer. I got the idea from a TV show called *Tim Gunn's Guide to Style*. Tim Gunn had a way of connecting with people, instructing with kindness and expertise that made him a well-loved television personality. Tim did one makeover per show for a nominated hot mess of a guest. He taught them to observe their body's shape objectively and to choose complimentary clothing by structure, garments built for their shape, fitting them together like puzzle pieces. He taught them to make clothing choices based on tangible criteria, instead of by emotion. Using simple techniques of pairing body shape with clothing styles, guests were transformed visually, and that process opened floodgates of self-acceptance they had never felt before or perhaps had lost along the way. I began to apply the principles to my own wardrobe, and my hopes soared. Perhaps I wasn't fundamentally flawed, perhaps the clothes I had been wearing were at fault. I had never known how to pick out clothes for myself.

Each episode reminded me there are a million reasons why women lose themselves in adulthood. I learned that not caring for our physical selves can be a symptom of a deeper struggle. Sometimes, as with me, it was as simple as not knowing how to choose the right clothing. Time and age and childbirth can change a woman's shape drastically, leaving us feeling as though we are living in a stranger's body. Frustration and disappointment at this betrayal can leave us feeling hopeless, embarrassed and ugly. Some women throw in the towel, allowing socially constructed ideals of feminine beauty to defeat them. It seems easier not to care. Abdicating care for one's physicality is tempting when every thread of life pulls at your center. Considerable effort is required to retain a sense of joy in your body, finding pleasure in caring for it and maintaining the pulse of sensuality, when every media message says that youth and beauty matter above all.

At the end of each show, guests had a big reveal moment. Every single episode ended with the entire cast weeping, including me. I watched faithfully, shedding tears on the couch as I saw the way these women felt about their new look, and the joy of their families when they saw their loved one give themselves the care and attention they deserved. The makeover guests had not lost weight or even been told to. They hadn't been told to look or act younger, or to wear clothes they were not comfortable in, but to embrace their very own selves. Each woman was transformed physically and emotionally. That's what I wanted, too.

At the same time, Tim Gunn was inspiring women, the US version of the BBC show *What Not to Wear* was taking off like wildfire. The premise of the series was the same, in that women were shown how to look their best, however, the hosts of *What Not to Wear* made snarky comments behind the guests' backs. There was less compassion involved, and I knew that less compassion was not what I needed. I doubted that anyone else did, either. Sadly, snarky won out, and Tim's show was canceled. Sarcasm gets better ratings. I was disappointed to know that the lack of compassion I aimed at myself was popular. However, I was on fire to learn these new skills for myself. This was personal, and I sought out the information I needed like a hound on the scent.

In the wake of the show's popularity, bookstores and websites abounded with how-tos for pairing clothing style with body structure, along with ideas about how to play with color and accessories, and I absorbed it all. The touted new "rules of style" appealed to my tendency to think linearly. Rules and formulas I understood. As I figured out what my body needed on the outside, I was able to look in the mirror without dismay for the first time. Self-love might have been a stretch, but acceptance grew, for sure. Approaching clothing with puzzle-solving objectivity deleted my frustration at my physical imperfections, reducing them to an equation that could be solved. As my own confidence grew, I realized it was possible that I might be reasonably attractive.

Right around this time, I met a woman at the gym. We had kids in the same class at school. She noticed I watched style shows while on the treadmill. A willowy redhead brimming with self-confidence, style, and artistic clothing was Annette's thing, while body acceptance and confronting insecurity was my current learning curve. We figured the two put together could be a powerful force. With some creativity and a bit of plagiarizing, we developed a curriculum designed to teach women to dress their shape. We wrote packets, instructions, and lists. We met clients for one-on-one style consultations at a local consignment shop and hosted style parties for groups of women; developed short episodes for the local TV channel and put on makeover shows as fundraisers for many different groups. I wrote film shorts that we had professionally produced and put on YouTube. I created a website with reviews of consignment shops from all over the region, as we focused on making style affordable for all. My newfound passion spilled over at home. I was excited about it and happy. I eagerly learned the computer skills required to manage it all.

"You're so independent now," Roger said to me one night, as he pulled the covers up to his chin. "It's like living with a different person."

He seemed out of sorts as if he wasn't quite sure what to do with me now. I felt as though I had, for the first time, found a skill that came naturally. When I shared the news of my new venture with Mom, I blurted out excitedly, "I'm good at it!"

"Oh, you are, are you?" she snapped sarcastically, and I remembered, self-confidence wasn't okay in her mind. I had forgotten.

"Yeah, I am," I responded before my throat could close, choking back the old familiar swell of shame I could no longer accept.

This was why I kept my distance from her. This was the thing I hoped I did not pass on to my own children. *Why was it so hard for her to be kind?* I wondered.

I never thought in a million years I could get up on a stage and speak a word, but when the opportunity came around, I did. I was passionate enough about my clients' transformations in the dressing room that I was willing to face the most paralyzing of all fears. Annette and I were the main performance at a women's event over the border at a church in British Columbia. Annette was a Christian, a topic of conversation we avoided and had made the connection to the group. We traveled to meet our makeover guest prior to the event, had gone through her wardrobe, and had taken her shopping. Her friends pitched in to have her hair and make-up done. When we presented her transformation onstage to her church community, she brought the house down. Annette and I beamed as the crowd applauded and whooped, and tears rolled down our guest's cheeks.

During the intermission, attendees had the opportunity to put style questions in a basket for us to answer in the last half of the show. The first question came to me.

"How do you get away with that color combination?" the slip of paper read. The tone was not friendly. My outfit of choice was a neon orange, paper-bag waist skirt (Calvin Klein clearance rack $5), a raspberry tee shirt (Target $8), a triple strand, silver chain necklace (thrift store $3) and bright, sky blue sling-back, high-heeled sandals (Nine West online clearance $35).

Annette sensed the confrontation in the question and, as an accomplished public speaker, attempted to intervene and soften the implied criticism, but I jumped right in with a smile.

"The short answer is I walked out the door, and nobody stopped me," I quipped with a grin.

The crowd of 300 erupted with laughter. I went on to explain the use of color blocking: pairing bright solids together, sans neutrals, in a single outfit without the distraction of patterns; and how the simplicity of this popular trend appealed to me, and the bright colors suit my complexion.

Then I shared, "I wore this outfit because it makes me happy and that is the whole point. No one has to approve of your reflection but you."

Again, the audience broke out into approving laughter and applause.

On the way home, after rehashing our successful evening, Annette asked how things were going at home. We had known each other a while at this point, and while we avoided talking about religion, we did talk about our husbands and kids. She knew I was not happy. I admitted that Roger and I were in dire straits and, if he continued to disengage from our marriage, I would have a decision to make.

As our business grew, I saw a lot of women in their underwear, which could have been weird, but wasn't. I was continually touched by the vulnerability and trust my clients exhibited in the dressing room with me. I found that I could meet a total stranger, and with acceptance and reliable information, my presence allowed them to be comfortable enough to change clothes in front of me. In the process, secrets came out. I heard about eating disorders, body shame, and insecurities, every bit of pain felt at being let down by self-perceived imperfections. I watched faces light up when they looked in the mirror exclaiming, "I would NEVER have picked this out for myself." Beautiful moments of smiles and tears as they gazed in wonder at their reflections gratified me and increased my love of the work.

My favorite service was closet makeovers, during which I hauled every last item of clothing my clients owned out into the light and reorganized their entire wardrobe, creating outfits they did not know they had. I showed them how to put combinations together themselves and to let go of unworn items. I wanted them to understand how to use clothing to reflect a renewed sense of self. The most effective way to reset style focus was to take a long hard look at their wardrobe and ask, "Who are you?" and "Who do you want to be?" I found that by showing my clients they were fine and beautiful and acceptable and worthy exactly how they were in that moment, my words echoed into my own heart, and I began to believe those things about myself. Together my clients and I found the courage to take a chance on ourselves, to be open about our doubts and fears. I also found a way to connect with other women, which I had never been able to do before.

I worked with several women who had lost 100 pounds or more, some after having had gastric bypass surgery. They always still saw the fat woman in the mirror. "Oh, I could never wear that size," they would say as I brought armloads of clothing into the dressing room. But they gamely tried the clothes on and were amazed. There was no better feeling for me than to watch smiles spread across their faces, replacing nervousness with joy, and to know that I never got it wrong.

After a few more months of sporadic client consultations, I had to face reality. While I dearly loved my work, there was no way to continue as a style consultant in a small town. The population base required to establish a steady income did not exist. The women I enjoyed working with the most were the ones without the confidence to call, making it difficult to connect. Annette was not interested in pursuing style consulting as a full-time job; she already had a career. I needed to work full time, but wasn't sure what to do next.

One of the last clients I worked with was a wealthy woman, a retired doctor's wife. She had several closets stuffed with unworn clothing. Every time I thought we were finished, she led me to another closet in another room, the last one packed with vintage St. John designer dresses worth thousands of dollars. After several hours of playing with her fabulous wardrobe, I gathered my things to go home.

"Just a minute," she said. "I want to show you something."

What now? I thought. I was starving and needed to pee.

She went back to her closet and knelt down, shoved some boxes aside, and slid open the cover of a hidden compartment in the wall. She pulled out a shoe box.

"When my son was in high school, his girlfriend had a baby who was put up for adoption," she said as she pulled out a handful of tattered snapshots. "No one knows I stayed in touch. This is my grandson."

I set my bag down on the floor and took the stack of photos of an infant, a toddler, a little boy. I was overwhelmed with the enormity of her secret and touched that she would share it with me. *What was it about this process that made her feel so safe? Why me?* I wondered.

She trusted me in her closet, even all the way to the back, where her deepest secret lay hidden. I wondered if the secrets looming in my own life and marriage would ever rise to the surface. I wondered what they were. I wondered where they were. I was honored that my clients felt safe with me, but I knew I did not feel safe in my own life. Changes were coming. Somehow this work was preparing me for whatever waited around the next corner.

Part Three

Chapter 14
Downward Spiral

Twenty years into a near-sexless marriage, I was quite literally going nuts from loneliness and desire. My body had been very busy with babies and exercise for years, fatigue keeping my desperation at bay. Pregnancy, childbirth, breastfeeding, diapers, finger-paint, goldfish crackers, repeat. Repeat, repeat, repeat. Daily exercise had been my habit for many years by this time, the intensity depending on my reproductive stage. I encouraged Roger to take care of himself, as well. He was a big guy, and I had always loved his muscles and size, but he had become increasingly obese. After one brief interlude of starving off all of his extra pounds, he looked fantastic, and our occasional sex was outstanding, at least by comparison. I could breathe in missionary position without being crushed by his gut. Our bodies fit together. He could run with his dog. He beamed at the constant compliments he received.

Once the weight was off, Roger set about eating the pounds back on. I watched from the kitchen sink as he sat down at the head of the dining room table with a plate of mashed potatoes and beef piled high. Again and again. In a fraction of the amount of time it had taken to lose seventy-five pounds, they all returned. I wondered if, like the physical barriers of boxes and filth that kept me out of his office, his obesity and slipshod personal hygiene were efforts to keep me away from his body. If so, the plan worked like a charm.

His office was an unfinished room accessible by walking through our closet. The walls were unpainted, the wooden floors missing slats. Dingy, white lace curtains left behind by the previous owners straggled across drafty windows. A U-shape of tables and desks housed Roger's banks of computers. Sliding piles of unopened mail, papers, and all variety of trash were strewn across every surface, layered with dust and grime. Every inch of the broken floor was piled with blank video cartridges, Star Trek models, empty boxes, and stuff. Emaciated cat shit caked with dust bunnies lay in the corners, and the cardboard boxes reeked of cat pee. Computer cords hung across the ceiling like wonky Christmas lights, dripping with cobwebs. There was a narrow path from the door to the desk chair. I did not go in there. The rest of the house was messy with kids and pets and one person picking up (me), but I managed to keep the chaos at bay everywhere else.

Roger and I turned in after the kids went to bed like we did every night. I climbed under the covers, pulling the quilt up over my hips. Roger swung the bedroom door shut, slipped off his bathrobe and hung it on the hook on the back of the door, a concession to my need for reasonable tidiness. As I watched him walk naked across the bedroom, I wanted to weep. His lack of self-care and disregard of his own health felt like a personal rejection. I wondered why he was going to such great lengths to keep me away from his body. I couldn't get anywhere near him. I worked hard at feeding the kids healthy food and staying fit myself. Why didn't he care?

As he climbed into bed beside me, the mattress rocked like a rowboat on a wave. I hung onto the edge until he and the bed had settled.

"Good night, love you," I said and reached over for a hug.

My fingers sunk into the rolls of fat around his middle. I recoiled and turned away to drift off to sleep on my side of the bed, with a desolate heart. The pressure was building. I was simultaneously repulsed by Roger while longing for his affection, yearning to be desired. I loved Roger. He said he loved me, but I couldn't feel it.

The next weekend, Roger and the kids cuddled up on the couch in the rec room to watch a sci-fi movie, as usual. They could always be found in a pile on the couch-Roger, kids, blankets, and dogs. I needed a break from the steady diet of aliens and laser beams and curled up alone in the other room to watch Comedy Central. A Jeff Foxworthy special was on. His "You might be a redneck if..." brand of comedy was popular in the early 2000s. He performed a bit about married sex, his point being that for all the travails of marriage, pleasuring his wife was like driving a familiar car. He knew where all the buttons were to rev her engine. My eyes filled with tears as I realized that after so many years, decades together, Roger had no idea how to bring me to orgasm. Something was terribly wrong. I clicked off the television and wandered in to join my family on the couch, sliding under the corner of a blanket and snuggling up next to the kid on the end.

I tried to focus on everything, anything, else but found myself shopping, buying more and more shoes online, the heels ever higher, for no good reason at all. I was running out of distractions and spending money we could not spare. One Saturday night, I was out with a group of soccer moms for drinks, listening to a local band play. The dance floor was hopping, and everyone was loose and happy. I saw Mike, one of the soccer dads, sitting alone on the other side of the bar. Mike and I had an electric connection; in group conversations, we always seemed to end up talking to each other. I bee-lined over to say hello and observed Mike bee-lining away from me. An almost audible voice in my head warned *do not follow*.

I halted, swerved, and went back to my table. There he was, buying everyone a round of drinks. I declined, knowing I was one beer away from foolish. We all hit the dance floor again, Mike and I were intensely aware of our proximity to each other. The band played oldies funk, the sensual thump and rhythm bounced through my body and moved my hips.

Back on our bar stools, sweaty and laughing, we couldn't take our eyes off each other. A woman I did not know asked us how long we had been together, which we denied with surprise.

"Mmmm, ok," she smirked, as she rolled her eyes and turned away.

He looked at me and confessed, "I am in love with you."

My heart stopped.

I laughed, "No, you're not, but that's a nice thing to say," pretending not to believe him.

I got the hell out of there as fast as possible. Emotional turmoil followed. He loved me? Did I love him? I wasn't sure, but I wanted him with teeth-rattling desire and decided an affair would be totally worth it. I wouldn't put him off again if another opportunity arose. How could this be happening? The internal acknowledgment of my own feelings terrified me. I was shaken to my core to admit I was willing to risk my marriage to sleep with Mike. I had never been unfaithful to Roger. A few men over the years flirted here and there, but I always shut them down without a second thought. Or at least without a third thought. Opportunities arose to stray over the course of our marriage, and I decided who I was in those moments. Faithful. That happens to everyone, right?

Mike and I never had another conversation. He began avoiding me like the plague. I got the message and tried to put him out of my mind. There was no way in hell I was going to cling to an inconvenient, unprovable fantasy about a man who wasn't coming for me. My insides were in pieces. There was no affair to run to, no romance to save me from doing the work required to fix my marriage. But I could no longer pretend to be happy. The truth of my misery had landed in my lap like a yowling wet cat. Leaving my marriage peacefully would have been a better choice at that point, but that was not the decision I made. I decided to do anything necessary to stay married and keep my family together. They say divorce is bad for kids and it is. What they don't say is having miserable parents is bad for kids, too.

I curled up on the overstuffed living room couch, sinking into the squishy pillows. Roger sat on the floor with the dog's head on his leg. I switched on the news so the kids wouldn't join us and turned to face him.

"Will you go to marriage counseling with me?" I asked.

Roger whirled around to look at me, surprise registering on his face.

"We don't have any problems we can't fix on our own," he answered, sounding shocked.

"Yeah, we do," I sighed. "I am going with or without you."

"Oh. Ok, I'll come," Roger agreed, then rose to his feet and left the room.

I attended the first counseling session alone. I shared my story of extra-marital attraction and my desire to find what was missing in my marriage. The therapist told me to feel my feelings.

"Learn to read your own body language," he said. "In moments of conflict, pay attention to where stress sits in your body. Those physical symptoms indicate what you are feeling. Acknowledge those feelings with words."

I could do that. I began to notice when my gut churned and burned, my chest tightened and my breath got shallow; when my pulse rose and cheeks flushed. I learned to observe those responses and track them back to what was happening at the moment, and then to identify and acknowledge the feelings behind them. I found out how often I felt ashamed and angry and sad. Often.

I noticed it when Roger interrupted and talked over me when I couldn't get my thoughts out fast enough. I noticed it when he stepped over me as I scrubbed the kitchen floor on my hands and knees, and stomped across the wet floor in his shoes. I noticed it when I was cooking and he took over, nudging me out of the way. I noticed it when I gave the kids a chore, and he told them they did not have to do it. I noticed my fuming silence. I was angry a lot.

Roger went to a counseling session alone, and then we went together. We were encouraged to meditate and talk to each other without accusation. Our communication improved immediately. I learned to speak without hurtling blame; Roger listened without defense. I knew I had to be honest with Roger about Mike if we were to continue to move forward. Mike felt like the elephant in the room.

Soon after, on a watery, spring Saturday afternoon, our whole family was at the soccer park, as usual. The kids had wandered off to their fields to warm up. Tournament season was upon us, and everyone had a game.

"I need to tell you something," I said to Roger as we strolled from the car toward the fields. "Sit with me?" I indicated a spot in the sun by the parking lot.

We lowered onto the slatted wooden bench, not touching or looking at each other. I shoved my hands in the pockets of my jacket and stretched out my legs, searching for the warmth of the sun.

"Mike told me he is in love with me," I confessed, conveniently leaving out my own willingness to have an affair.

I looked over at Roger. He sat with his eyes closed, hands clasped over his stomach, breathing deeply, as our therapist had instructed him to do during meditation.

"Ok," he said.

"Nothing happened. He didn't touch me or anything," I continued.

"Are you in love with him?" Roger asked.

"Well... attracted, for sure," I evaded, still protecting myself.

Roger did not respond.

We sat in silence in the weak sunlight. Familiar families walked past, with a smile and a wave. I smiled back, lips in a tight grimace, an attempt at normalcy. I saw their smiles falter as they walked away, sensing the tension. Roger and I gathered ourselves and walked through the wet grass for the first game of the day in silence.

The following week was quiet as we tiptoed around each other. Money was too tight to continue marriage counseling, so I canceled our next appointment. We were more disconnected than ever. For me, the main thing missing from our relationship was sex. I still did not know why Roger did not want me, but I wanted to try to want him. I was fit, horny, and as attractive as it was possible for me to be. Why couldn't he join me?

A few summers before, I sat in our filthy minivan with my mother in law, Beth, and my youngest child, Oliver, who was still a baby. We were headed home from a camping trip on Lopez Island while the rest of the family sailed back to Bellingham on a borrowed boat. Beth asked me to pull over at Farm to Market Bakery in Bow. Oliver slept in his car seat while she ran in, returning with a gooey strawberry Danish. I was shocked to see the pastry in her hand. Beth never ate in front of anyone.

"We're so glad Roger found you; you're good for him. Jerome and I just love you for him," she smacked glaze from her fingers. "We always wondered if maybe he was gay."

My stomach dropped.

"Do you want half?" she asked, holding out the pastry, butter spreading onto the brown paper napkin.

"No, thank you," I muttered as I pulled out onto Bow-Edison Road toward Chuckanut Mountain.

I had sometimes wondered if Roger might be gay, and so had my sister. I had broached the subject of his possible homosexuality in the past a few times, but he always disregarded me. He never vehemently denied it, just kinda, sorta said he wasn't, somehow. I certainly did not want it to be true, what with four kids and a mortgage. I had no college education or career to fall back on, no way of supporting myself and the kids without him, which made me inclined to cling to any other possibility. Also, to hide his homosexuality from me after the way my father had handled his own coming out would be the most profound cruelty. Dad's lies had ransacked my family and broken my mother's heart. Roger loved me too much to do that. Didn't he?

I did not think Roger was cheating on me since he rarely left the house. We had partnership habits grounded in the comfortable patterns of family life. Companionship can feel a lot like love. Maybe we just needed to try harder.

In order to close the sex gap, I began to research open marriage and sex positivity, looking for a solution. I read *Open* by Jenny Block and *Mating in Captivity* by Esther Perel, *Sex at Dawn* by Christopher Ryan and anything by Betty Dodson and Dan Savage. I became convinced that opening our marriage to other sexual partners was the answer to staying together, a way to hold onto my last shred of sanity. I could have devoured an entire adult male with my vagina at that point. Extended lack of physical attention feels like starving. And madness.

While perusing articles online, I discovered an education-centered, sex-positive website and after downloading a short instructional video, a message from a sex coach popped up in my email. He offered one free thirty-minute introductory phone call with the opportunity to sign up for coaching sessions afterward. I signed up on the spot.

After some emails back and forth, the sex coach and I arranged a call for the following day, and I made sure Roger knew to keep the kids out of my office. I sat at my desk watching my phone, a pad of paper and pen ready for note-taking. My heart thumped with excitement. The sex coach called right on time.

"Why are you interested in sex coaching? Tell me about your situation," he asked. His friendly, professional voice put me at ease.

"My husband and I are sexually disconnected. I'm looking for ways to spice things up. I need more. And I am interested in opening our marriage to other partners, as well," I said honestly.

"Whoa, one step at a time. Opening a marriage can present difficulties. Let's focus on reconnecting you two to each other first," he wisely suggested. "Got your pen ready?"

I learned more in that thirty-minute conversation than I ever had about sexual communication. I couldn't take notes fast enough. The coach described, in specific detail, a variety of positions for us to try, effectively creating a to-do list for the bedroom. I felt as though I had been given a treasure map to find the magic kingdom of marital bliss. In reality, having specific positions to try forced Roger and me to touch each other, which was a good way to find out if we wanted to.

The most important message from the free session was the coach's instruction to approach sexual exploration as practice. We should proceed with the understanding that we were trying out something new, the same way you would try out a recipe. Perhaps we would like the new position, perhaps not. No pressure, no expectations. Let it be relaxed, maybe even funny. No one had to be the expert. If a position did not feel good, we were to scratch it off the list. This way of thinking effectively deleted any performance anxiety. The positions themselves mattered very little but provided tangible ways to start exploring. What I did not realize was that we were not addressing the problem.

Despite being financially strapped, we signed up for sessions with the sex coach, three for me, three for Roger, including written responses after trying new positions. The sessions seemed like a good investment, just the thing to fix us up, and a more direct approach than therapy.

We tried the new positions once each; checking them off the list like chores. We had some satisfying sexual experiences during that time, as well as some failures. We seemed to be making progress and got good grades from the sex coach. The coach neglected to take notes to move our progress along and thus repeated himself and started over at every meeting. He did not remember what he had covered and what he hadn't; did not remember what we had said was off the table (anal, because you're wondering). He had shared his best information in the free phone call. While he had a long way to go in terms of professionalism, the experience did prove valuable. Learning to approach sex without expectation was freeing. Also, I got a vibrator and bright blue rubber dildo with the deal. My firsts.

I know now what was missing, now that I have it. The holding, the soaking each other up with hands on skin and the gaze of loving eyes, the wanting. Freda Kahlo said, "Take a lover who looks at you as if maybe you are magic." Roger and I had never had that. Perhaps neither of us ever had with anyone. Our experiment fell flat once the positions on the list were marked off.

Then Roger gave me a fancy vibrator for Christmas. The wrapped package was waiting for me on my pillow when we turned in after a long, full day. I shook the vibrator out of the box, tissue paper strewn on the floor by the bed. A two-pronged green Lelo, smooth as silk to the touch, lay inside. I was delighted by this sweet, romantic gesture, an acknowledgment of my needs. The vibrator was pretty complicated, with a lot of lights and buttons. We crawled into bed and, as I attempted to navigate the controls, Roger shut off his nightlight, rolled over, pulled the blanket up over his shoulder, and went to sleep. He had thrown the dog a bone, and he was done.

I carried on alone, holding the vibrator up under the blanket, trying to figure out the controls by the light of the "ON" button. Finally, it roared to life like a Harley. I tentatively touched it to myself and jumped, the sensation akin to an electric shock. I am not certain of its horsepower, but I'm pretty sure it could have pulled the Wells Fargo wagon. I gingerly touched the wand to my clit again. The Lelo provided too much stimulation at first, but not for long. I orgasmed alone and went to sleep.

I began to push the idea of open marriage with Roger, in a last ditch effort to get ethically laid. There did not seem to be any other alternative. Despite my newfound love of vibrators, I needed a man. I wanted my husband to want me, and if he couldn't, then someone else would do. With twenty years, four kids and tenuous finances, splitting up seemed unthinkable. Divorce was not even on the table; we never discussed it at all.

I know now that open relationships work when a mutual decision is made, born of the desires of both partners. When the decision to open a relationship is made because one person is unhappy, failure is inevitable. We failed on an epic scale. Roger refused to read anything about how to responsibly open our marriage, although he agreed to the concept in theory. I brought the subject up, again, in the kitchen one afternoon as we stood at opposite ends of the island. He stared out the window as I pestered for freedom.

"Ok, do whatever you have to do to be happy," he sighed sadly.

I turned around, walked through my office door, shutting it firmly behind me. I sat down at my computer and turned it on with no real idea of what to do next.

Chapter 15
Hustle

We did not have any money. While visiting family over the Christmas holidays I admitted to my sisters that we were going home to empty cupboards with no way to fill them. We were busted. They both slipped me some cash, for which I was embarrassed and grateful. I knew I had to find a real job, which meant that our home life would go to hell, nothing would ever be clean again, and it was only a matter of time before my adolescent children were left in the rain and squirrels were living in the kitchen, but there was no choice. I had taken on several part-time jobs in addition to sporadic style consulting: census taker, consignment shop person, dental office receptionist, none of which provided enough income or stability. I was always seeking a way to increase our income and still be available to the kids, but now I needed something full time and permanent to keep the family afloat. It was up to me.

A friend gave me the number of a psychotherapist named Geri who managed a group of mental health providers and was looking for office help. I called her right away, several times, but got no response. I took a deep breath and left one more message. Geri called back this time and asked me to come in right away for an interview. She seemed pretty frazzled on the phone.

We met at her peacefully appointed counseling office overlooking Bellingham Bay on a Sunday afternoon and chatted for a few minutes while I tried not to act desperate. The serenity of her office, with its sage green walls and soft lighting, belied the stress in her eyes. Geri explained that ten mental health providers shared a central staff. She was the administrative manager, as well as one of the providers. Things were not going well, administratively speaking. She led me across the hall into the haphazard central office and turned on one of the computers. The L-shaped room was crammed with desks and tables, each awash with monitors, file folders, and piles of stuff. The mess was a little familiar.

"Let me show you our new software system," she said, fumbling with her password.

The program came online after a few tries. Watching Geri attempt to navigate the medical office management software system was like reading a language I did not know I knew. I could see it was foreign to her, but I understood it. I stopped myself from telling her how to use the program as I watched over her shoulder, and tried to nod and smile.

I started the next day.

All ten psychiatrists, psychologists, and therapists had been without regular staff for three months. The previous office manager had been fired under mysterious circumstances at the beginning of the year; no one said why. On that same day, the other office administrator quit. Now it was April. No one knew how to use the new software system. Ten full-time providers translate to at least 500 patients and clients per week, in and out the door. After three months with no staff, there were approximately 6,000 appointments to be billed and/or rebilled, each one needed to be sorted out individually. 6,000 appointments worth of copayments, insurance claims and reimbursements, all in sliding piles of manila folders stuffed with cash, checks, and credit card slips. Unposted payments, many unidentifiable, were stacked everywhere. Most insurance claims had not been submitted or had been filed incorrectly. Tens of thousands of dollars of insurance reimbursements were missing. Folders were tucked in cupboards and bins and hidden in Geri's office. Doctors accustomed to making a quarter of a million dollars a year or more could not pay their mortgages. Geri continually reassured them that she had everything under control; that it was a matter of a few more days until things were straightened out. Her reassurances were patently false. Patients were infuriated that their checks were uncashed, payments unaccounted for, and insurance claims un-submitted, leaving their deductibles unmet. Chaos reigned.

I sat down in a sagging wicker kitchen chair in the back corner of the office on my first morning and tentatively took a stack of folders, slid the top one onto my desk and flipped it open. The former employee who had previously resigned stopped by for an hour to give a quick lesson in claims submission on the new system, a process she had been shown once. I took furious notes. The software company had a very patient support technician upon whom I relied. A few months later, after speaking with me multiple times a day, she quit. Not my fault, I hope.

Brooke, who came in once a week to make deposits, stopped by my desk and leaned over to whisper, "Hide everything you are working on before you leave at night. Geri will go through your desk after you go home. She moves stuff around, and sometimes she takes things. She can't leave anything alone. If she takes your work into her office, you'll never see it again."

"Thank you," I gasped in horror, eyes wide. *What have I gotten myself into?* I wondered.

"You're welcome," she whispered with an apologetic smile, shuffling off with her arms full of folders, deposit slips, and calculators.

My presence as a surprise new staff member was duly noted by the physicians. Dr. Jacobs stood in the middle of the office with a blank, panicked look, his eyeballs quivering as he stared at me. The thought bubble over his head clearly stated, *"Who the hell is this?"* He did not introduce himself or utter a word. After a moment, he turned away, walked into his office, and shut the door. I did not see him again for the rest of the day.

I returned my attention to the computer and navigated my way into the system, which was remarkably easy to use, intuitive. This was a huge relief since I had presented myself as being far more experienced than I was. A few weeks spent answering the phone in a dental office where I was not allowed to touch anything to do with insurance was all the billing experience I had. I had seen insurance forms on the dentist's wife's pile of papers. Upside down, from the other side of the desk. That was about it. I soon realized medical billing was all Sudoku; arranging numbers in boxes. Put the right number in the right box, and everything works. Persistence was required, but it was not rocket science. And I love Sudoku.

Mid-way through the first morning, Dr. McCoy, another one of the psychiatrists, typed up a half page note protesting the presence of new and unknown staff, naming me personally, along with Mary, the other new hire. Dr. McCoy shoved her vitriolic slips of paper into each of the other doctors' inboxes, complaining to Geri in full speed jabber. Her flyaway hair seemed upset, too. I wasn't really listening; there was too much work to do. I had already been working for several hours from the sagging seat of that ancient kitchen chair and my back already hurt, so was in no mood for harassment. Also, I knew this doctor. Our sons played on the same indoor soccer team. I swiped a copy of her note out of one of the doctor's inboxes when no one was looking and read it:

Dear Providers,

We have two new people in the office, Mary and Rona. We have been given no references and no information re: who they are. We do not know if they have any experience or are trustworthy. I have a problem with people being hired sight unseen and would like to call an emergency meeting of all members.

I handed the note to Dr. McCoy when she came back into the office.

"Hi, I'm Ronna. My name is spelled with two Ns," I said, pointing to her misspelling. "Our sons play soccer together."

She blanched, her cheeks turned white under her freckles. She whirled around and went back to her office without a word, taking her note with her.

I got back to work. There was no way in hell this doctor's tantrum was going to jeopardize my paycheck. I had kids to feed. I observed that Mary was still on Facebook, where she would remain until the day she quit.

Thirteen hours later, my back screaming now, I went home. I had made $169 before taxes. Supporting a family of six on $13 an hour did not seem possible, but the money would help, and I had to start somewhere. When I got home, I inhaled leftover spaghetti over the kitchen sink and collapsed into bed. I got up the next morning and did it again. And again.

I began to walk to work after our second car died to leave the minivan with Roger. He was in charge of chauffeuring kids now. Leaving for work early to get to the office before the deluge of patients, ringing telephones and providers descended, I walked the Sehome Hill Arboretum trail in the dark to the Western Washington University. Wooden steps from the dirt trail descended to sidewalks that swept past the beautiful brick building of Old Main, and through the deserted campus, sculptures wet and still in the light of the street lamps, to a dead end neighborhood street. At the curve of the dead-end street, I caught another trail that cut through a wooded area called Lowell Park. The path through Lowell Park forest let out at the top of Taylor Street. From there it was a short jog over to Knox Avenue and down the hill to the office. From the top of Knox, Bellingham Bay stretched out before me in the dawn, soft harbor lights reflecting on the still water. The path became a meditation, my mind blissfully free as I walked the familiar route in silence.

I walked the path every day, in every weather. One pitch black morning, as I picked my way through the woods of Lowell Park, something hit me on top of the head with enormous force. My knees buckled. I grabbed the top of my head, gasping in pain. Had I run into a low hanging branch? There hadn't been one over the trail the day before, and we hadn't had any high winds. I stopped to look around, my eyes adjusting to the dark as I clutched my scalp, breathing heavily.

Off to the right, a large owl sat on a branch, watching me steadily as if to say, "What are you doing here?" *Those were owl talons bashing my skull in,* I thought. *What the fuck? They felt like lead.* I stared back at the owl. Lowell Park was its territory, and I was trespassing. *Better keep moving,* I thought.

I continued on to work, holding onto my aching head, hoping I wasn't bleeding all over the place and deep breathing to manage the pain. When I got to the office bathroom, I saw there was a small, slightly bloody dent in the top of my throbbing scalp. I rubbed hand sanitizer into it. Woozy and headachy, I sat down in my chair at the back of the office and worked my way through another stack of slip-sliding file folders. I did not think to ask any of the doctors in the building to check my pupils for signs of a concussion. If the owl had knocked my head any harder, I could have lost consciousness, and it would have been the sole witness. How long would I have lain in the dirt before anyone found me? Quite a while, I surmised.

As I settled into the job, work became an escape from the realities of my marriage and home. I was relieved to be up to my eyeballs with numbers to line up in boxes, black and white problems with specific solutions. A calmness descended when confronted by mountains of medical billing. Number arranging was just the thing to distract me. Unlike my disintegrating home life, this was something I could fix. The responsibility of employment allowed me to check out of the family every morning and think about something else.

The following months were a blur. I had no idea what my children were doing, no idea how any of us survived. I worked, and I worked. Sheer force of will kept me together. Chaos reigned at home when I had time to notice. The house was filthy, the cupboards bare, as I knew they would be. My children were neglected, and Roger and I seldom spoke. Still, my body's need for touch felt like a pounding pulse.

I got home after another long workday, to find Marie crying in the window seat.

"You work ALL THE TIME," she sobbed. Roger had forgotten to pick her up at soccer practice.

What could I say? I sat down next to her, wrapping my arms around her little body.

"I know, sweetie," I said. "I have to. I'm so sorry." I kissed her blond head, breathing in the sweet candy smell of her silky hair, swallowing my own tears.

I stumbled into the kitchen where Roger was cooking, spaghetti again. I was starving and sad and furious.

"Hey, next time you're at Trader Joe's could you get some of that...," Roger began.

"WHAT?" I interrupted. "Whaddya mean, the next time I'm at Trader Joe's," I snapped, grabbing the pasta spoon. "You're home all day. YOU GO TO TRADER JOE'S."

His expression froze, and he did not respond.

I loaded a plate and went to the dining room where Jane sat at the table with her homework. "Oh my God, Mom, this house is FILTHY!" she accused, on the verge of tears of frustration. "It's embarrassing. I can't bring any of my friends over anymore. It's DISGUSTING!"

"Well, maybe you should help out. This is not MY mess. I'm at work all day. Maybe the people who are here all day making the mess could CLEAN IT UP!" I yelled, slapping my plate on the table. Jane's jaw set in anger as she returned her attention to her homework.

After I finished the dishes, Roger and I stood in the kitchen, at opposite ends of the island. My monthly paycheck covered the mortgage, but nothing else, and Roger was not bringing in any income at all. We had just eaten the last bag of pasta.

"Roger, you have to get a job," I pleaded. "You have to do something. Apply to Fred Meyers or Costco. I heard WTA is hiring drivers. Do something. *Anything*. Please."

"If I get a job, I'll just have to quit when my show sells," he countered uneasily, shifting his weight.

"So what? So you'll quit. You have to do something to get us through," I reasoned impatiently, exasperated, desperate.

"That wouldn't be fair to an employer," he wheedled.

"WE DON'T HAVE ANY FOOD," I spat.

He squirmed and shifted his weight from foot to foot, turned and disappeared into his office. All of my fears regarding his unwillingness to take care of us came crashing in as he walked away. He was never going to help.

An hour or so later, he came up with a few hundred dollars for groceries. I did not know where the money came from. When I asked, he said it was from the business account. His answer was vague, evasive, but I figured if I pushed he would lie, so there was no point pressing. At least we would have something to eat.

I went back to work. Every time I got to the bottom of a stack of file folders, another appeared on my desk. When the stacks were finally finished, Geri pulled out an enormous blue plastic storage bin from under a table in the corner.

"These should be looked into, probably," she muttered, attempting to shove it across the floor in my direction.

I peeled off the lid to discover stacks of rubber-banded bundles of old claims. I sighed and dug in.

When my co-worker Mary wasn't around, I scrolled through the billing reports for the provider accounts assigned to her. Nothing was done. I wondered how she had so much time for Facebook; she was not doing the work. I discovered she posted false payments to make it appear that claims were paid when they were not. She had not tackled the backlog of work at all, instead created false entries to make it appear as though she had.

With so much of the work seemingly caught up, Mary's assigned doctors were still missing tens of thousands of dollars in income. This was why. She was faking it. *So that's where the money was going*, I thought. *Now it makes sense.*

I sat Geri down with the evidence. "Mary is faking the books. If all this work is going to end up in my lap anyway, please tell me now so I can get started."

"Ummm, I don't know..." she said as she looked away, apparently unwilling to have the confrontation.

When the day came, not long after, that Mary walked out leaving mountains of work in her wake, I presented a demand for a significant wage increase. My request was honored on the spot. I turned back to my screen and proceeded to complete the unfinished work with a sigh of relief. I had attained a stable job at an almost-but-not-quite livable wage.

I was still horny and unsatisfied and more emotionally alone than ever. If it was up to me to support my family and get myself laid, so be it. I was done waiting for salvation.

By the time Roger and I agreed to an open relationship, we had already stopped having sex with each other, no longer bothering to pretend. I was relieved to stop trying, but the idea of venturing out was daunting. How? Where? With whom? All possibilities seemed like a recipe for disaster. The concept of online philandering was frightening. I had no idea how to protect myself and did not want to end up strangled by a stranger in a shitty hotel room. Going insane from lack of physical contact did not seem like a good idea, either, and I was more than halfway there already.

At Temple Bar with T, over cocktails. She suggested I peruse Craigslist for a hook-up and walked me through how to seek partners safely. Be clear that you don't want a relationship. Be specific about what you are looking for. Meet in a public place first. Above all, trust your instincts. She was reassuring, encouraging and kind. "You can do it, just be careful," she said. "Know what you want."

Shut away in my office at home, I googled sex sites, unwilling to start with Craigslist. There had to be a way to ease in without having to meet someone in the food court at the mall. Up popped an appropriately slutty website in about half a second. Triple X seemed like just the thing. The profile template offered complete anonymity and a multitude of lists for specificity. I could window shop as long as I wanted. I checked off the boxes:

Likes: red wine

Looking for: male

No: overweight, over 60

Yes: check all

I took a selfie of a chest shot in my closet; soft light, teal silk camisole, hard nipples. *Not bad,* I thought, *sexy but not skanky and utterly unidentifiable.*

Here goes, I thought as I pressed Publish Profile. Email messages popped up within minutes. I turned on the instant messaging function. Digital floodgates opened and my screen filled with message bubbles, far too many to read. I turned IM off, overwhelmed, feeling as if I had accidentally opened a hatch to the underworld. There were a shocking number of men online. Even though my profile was specific about my "Nos," men did not pay attention to what I did not want. Males from twenty to eighty years of age asked to meet. I received an offer of a come shot to the face by way of introduction and wondered if that person ever got a positive response. An angry middle-aged man sought young females in Catholic school girl uniforms. A skinny kid wanted a MILF experience, and an eighty year old with a sailor's hat and pipe reassured me that he could still get hard. A buff, happy looking dude who referred to himself as Alley Cat professed to be allowed to play by an understanding partner like I was. Not all of them were married. The ones that confused me were the men with girlfriends. Trapped and married I understood, but if they were not legally committed, couldn't they just break up? Perhaps it was not that simple.

I changed my parameters, just for fun, to check out the competition. What kinds of women were on sex sites? I pretended to be a man looking for a woman. There were no others like me on the site, at least not in the area: one very young woman seeking an older companion, a couple seeking a third and someone who wrote and posted her own fantasy stories. ("She sank onto his mighty python…")

Hoo, boy, I'm golden. I thought as I scrolled. I could take my time to pick and choose without revealing myself. Being desired by so many men was intoxicating, as was the opportunity to peruse them as if they were cats in a cardboard box.

Before I got my profile completed, a hot bodybuilder named Rob emailed me, "Where's your picture, hun?" Somehow there was something sweet and laid back about the tone. His body had my attention. We chatted for a while through the website email.

Rob would say, "Come fuck me."

Rob would say, "How soon can I get you on my cock? I want to fuck you right now. Do you want some ass? Be honest…"

Somehow when he said it, it was charming and funny, and I just wanted to do it. And he WAS charming and funny. We met once, but he wouldn't wear a condom because he couldn't stay erect in one. He masturbated in the back seat of my car, and we said good-bye. He said he did not play around much, but who was he kidding? He continued to send messages for a while, "Baby, I want to see you again." I laughed and thought about it for a second, but I did not answer.

Then there was Ben. Sweet, sad Ben.

I waited in line for him at Starbucks. At the back of the coffee shop, I saw a familiar face, a woman from the gym who had recently divorced and looked to be on a date. I hovered behind other customers hoping she wouldn't spot me until Ben walked in. Thirty years old, semi-professional football player, an enormous man, and completely hairless, with the fattest cock I had ever seen in my life. He could bench over 400 pounds and had bullet scars from getting caught in gang crossfire while growing up in Detroit. He seemed to need a hug and a friend more than a lover and probably had PTSD.

He did not make much eye contact as he mumbled, "Let's get out of here." He had walked, so we drove together back to his condo. I was sweating, driving down Northwest Avenue, wondering how I would explain being seen with this hulking man in my minivan. As we pulled into his parking lot, he described being mugged on the sidewalk outside his building. I gulped, wondering what kind of neighborhood this guy could get mugged in. He showed me into his place, and I was awed. Clean white walls soared to the second story, showcasing gorgeous black and white framed photography of Muhammed Ali and other athletes.

We walked upstairs to his open loft bedroom and began to undress, somewhat awkwardly. Neither of us knew how to ask for what we wanted. As we touched and kissed, he became quickly and fearsomely erect. He rolled on a condom and turned me over to my hands and knees with his giant hands. He began thrusting, bang, bang, bang.

"What are you doing?" I asked after a minute. He seemed to be working so hard.

"I'm trying to make you come," he said.

"Umm, well... let's try something else," I proposed, easing out from underneath him.

The magnum condom had shredded on his too-large penis. It was almost a relief to give up. We masturbated side by side, and I never saw him again. I hope he found someone.

Marc kept popping up as a good match for me. His black and white profile photograph looked like a dating site advertisement; a little too sweet, a little too nice-guy. Most of the pictures on Triple X were lousy, ill-lit, surreptitious phone snaps. Or dick pics. Marc emailed, and I decided to meet him after some pleasant exchanges. He was receptive and sociable, normal-ish.

We met at a café by my office for tea. He was quiet and reserved. We sat, tucked away, at a little table in the corner.

"Do you like cunnilingus?" Marc asked politely.

I giggled to myself, having never heard the word cunnilingus uttered out loud before.

"Erm, yes, I do. Thanks for asking," I smiled.

After ordering, I looked around at the other diners and laughed. The surrounding tables seemed very close.

"I wonder what *they're* talking about," I grinned, keeping my voice low.

Marc did not laugh. He had no discernible sense of humor. He explained that after his divorce, his job had taken him to South America for several months where he met a hot local girlfriend he was loathed to leave behind. She had begged to have his babies, he said. I found it disconcerting to compete with a tropical, fertile, free-spirited beauty half my age who may or may not be real. Despite his high standards, he invited me to his condo, which was thirty seconds from my office in the other direction.

I stopped by after work, as planned. The door opened, and Marc invited me in, somewhat hesitantly. I walked in with confidence and moved right in with a hug. I wasn't there to get to know him. Marc stepped away from me, uncomfortable. He wanted to map out our session first. *Hmmm... you mean like make a list?* I wondered. I thought we had done that over tea. (Cunnilingus, yes; anal, no; condoms, absolutely.) We settled onto his white leather couch. I reached out a hand to his leg. He recoiled.

"Let's wait until we get to bed," he said.

Things seemed to go pretty well once we got there. Marc was skilled with hands and tongue, eliciting immediate tingles, but then, oh my God. He had the hardest penis I had ever felt. Oddly, strangely, uncommonly hard. T told me later that he must have been on Viagra. He couldn't come. At all. Never did. His abnormally hard penis was angled so that it jackhammered right into my G-spot, but not in a good way.

As he fucked me doggie-style, I thought I was going to hit the wall with my face, hanging onto fistfuls of sheets yelling, "FUCK, oh God, please come."

But no.

And what is it with doggie-style, anyway?

I ended up getting myself off, alone, again.

Afterward, we lay back on his pillows.

"I can either come right away or not at all," he said by way of explanation, his penis still like granite.

"Huh. Ok," I muttered, searching the sheets for my underwear.

Something was not working for Marc, though, because on the way out the door his schedule became full.

"I'll wait to hear from you," I said, knowing he wouldn't call. And he did not. I must admit to a moment or two of insecurity. Is my stretched out stomach skin that much of a turn-off? Am I that bad at sex? What happened next threw those insecurities right out the window. Then I met Vlad.

Chapter 16
Grit

Back at Temple Bar with T, mulling over our experiences of having sex with strangers. She looked out the window, not meeting my gaze. Turning her cocktail on its napkin. She told me her roommate had shown her a profile picture on a gay website of someone they thought looked like Roger.

"Is that happening?" she asked.

My heart landed in the pit of my stomach with an almost audible thud.

I remembered a conversation with Roger from the day before yesterday as I sat cross-legged on our bed. He stood in the doorway to the closet, inching toward the door. We were discussing his upcoming tryst with a woman he met online. He had a date planned to meet her at a bar. Her husband would be there, also.

"So her husband is coming, too?" I queried.

"Yeah, I guess they check out her partners together first," he responded uneasily.

"Does the husband join in? Is this going to be a threesome?" I pushed.

"I don't know," Roger admitted, shifting his weight from foot to foot.

"What if he does? What are you going to do?" I asked, an edge of panic tinging inside my head. "Are you okay with that?"

"Please say no, please say you'll walk away if her husband wants to touch you. Please, please don't want him to," I begged internally, my stomach knotted.

"Oh, well you know, it doesn't matter who's down there if you close your eyes," Roger blushed bright red, waving his hand at me as he turned and fled into his office and shut the door. I did not have the courage to follow, sat glued to the bed, paralyzed by what his evasiveness might mean. I needed the absolute truth but was too scared to demand it.

I watched T's expression in the reflection of the bar window as she gazed out at the dark street, avoiding eye contact with me. I could hardly breathe, knowing in my gut it was Roger. He was on gay websites. How many times had I opened the door to that conversation? How many times had I said the words, offering him the opportunity to be honest, to tell me his truth, to break me gently? He must know this was the one thing I couldn't handle; that this would destroy me, and would end us. He had to know that.

"I don't know if he's doing that or not," I shrugged and downed my Salty Dog. "I better get home for dinner."

My heart thudded in my chest as I walked toward my car. My heart was the only thing I could hear. I moved through the house, numb. Dinner made it to the table, the kids chattered around me, ate, and dispersed, as if in a dream once removed. My head pounded.

Afterward, I stood at the kitchen sink, hands in hot, soapy dishwater. Roger sat at the table, watching.

"T said they saw someone who looks like you on a website her roommate cruises." I ventured carefully. "Was it you?"

Roger knew T's roommate was gay; he understood the implication.

"Ahhhh, I don't know. What site?" he shrugged, feigning nonchalance.

I held his gaze a moment.

"I don't know which one," I turned away to wipe down the counters.

Well, that wasn't a no. The next question could only be what gay websites are you on? I couldn't ask it. The silence pulsed. Roger vanished into his office.

Later still, kids asleep, Roger and I crawled into bed on our respective sides, the same sides we had slept on for twenty-two years as if a motion trigger bomb sat in the middle of the mattress. I lay with my back to Roger at the edge of the bed, body tense in the darkened room, filtered moonlight gleamed off the brass bedposts.

"Was it you?" I asked, gazing at the shadows on the wall.

"Yes," he answered.

As if controlled by an outside force, my body levitated and whirled around, my right hand raised and hit Roger as hard as possible in the face. He did not see it coming in the dark. When I came back into my body, I had already started to scream. I re-entered myself in mid-shriek. Voltage from my lungs, my words hurled through the room.

"You're fucking gay? You lied, you lied, YOU LIED! HOW DARE YOU LIE TO ME ABOUT THAT? I had a right to know. I want a divorce. I want my twenty years back," I howled.

I was up, we were up, grabbing for robes. Lights on, twenty years of rejection, confusion, and fear erupted in uncontrolled ten-decibel rage. I was terrifying, insane, nothing-will-ever-be-the-same-again furious. The fantasy of our happiness was permanently shattered.

Twenty years of being shut out, of timidly knocking on the door to his heart, to his body; denied access. Twenty years of asking, of questioning myself, of wondering what was wrong, of wondering what was wrong with me. How could he do this to me?

I had snapped. My mind was blank. I hardly knew what was spewing out of my mouth.

The kids were up, seventeen-year-old Jane stood between us. "There are children in the house!" she yelled, not counting herself. Brutus, the Yorkie-poo, ran around the room, whining. Marie and Oliver stood sobbing in the hall.

I stopped screaming and saw my traumatized children standing around me. I heard the terrified dog. What had I done?

I stepped toward Marie.

"No, no," she said.

Stay away from me is what she meant. I'm scared of you is what she meant.

Somehow, we all made it downstairs, arranged on the couches and chairs. Alex showed up at the front door, walked in and pulled a dining room chair to the circle, as if at the head of the table. Jane had texted him to come home, and he did. He took over with calm, flat anger, the voice of reason, quietly blaming me for the situation, for my anger. Why I was mad did not matter to the kids. Roger, as the well-established fun parent, had their loyalty. Roger protected himself and lied, even then, even in that stark reality, vindicated that I had lost my temper while he remained calm; the sympathetic parent. This was not his fault; it was mine.

Uneasy quiet descended; there was nothing left to say. Alex left, and Roger and the kids went upstairs to bed. I stretched out on the couch for a sleepless night, staring at the darkened family room until I could get up and escape.

I went to work earlier than usual but did not say a word to anyone about the night before. After putting in eight hours at my desk in a blur of clarity and fury, I went home.

"I'm going to move into my office downstairs," I told Roger. "Can you please help me move the extra twin bed?"

We navigated the wooden frame down the stairs and set it up against the outside wall, stacked the mattress on top and found some extra blankets. My office, a beautiful room I designed myself, was my sanctuary. The one always-clean, no-pets-allowed room in the house, with mustard yellow walls, plush gray carpet, and a crystal chandelier. The place where kids could lay on the floor and have some peace. Now it was my home. It was also cold and drafty, the single pane windows poor defense against the wind. I would have to keep the blinds drawn to hold in any heat at all.

I went to work every day as usual and kept paying the mortgage. The kids wanted me to move out of the house since I wanted the divorce. Since I lost my temper and broke the spell of our family. Blame pointed in my direction like switchblades. The crushing vice of guilt twisted my gut.

I checked out the rental house across the alley. The rent was more than I could afford, but perhaps I could find a roommate. The kids would be able to run back and forth from house to house if they wanted to. I would be close, in case they wanted me to be. I walked back home, lease in hand, to discuss the arrangement with Roger. I found him in the kitchen.

"I'm going back to California. I can't stay here," he announced, from his end of the island in the kitchen.

"What are you talking about? I just rented the house across the alley," I responded angrily, from my end.

Blank stare.

"We can't both leave," I snapped. "We decided I was moving out, remember?"

Blank stare.

I backed out of the rental agreement, but then Roger did not pack his bags and leave. He stayed. He continued sleeping in the master bedroom, while I remained holed up in my office.

"When are you leaving?" I asked a week later, as I saw no indication that he was preparing to move.

"Well, I can't go now," he whined, "I can't afford to."

"Then you have to move out," I insisted. "I gave up the rental house because you said you were leaving, so leave."

"I'm going to stay here until I can afford to go. You can have the bedroom, and I'll move a bed into my office and use the back stairwell to come and go. The house is big enough for us both to live here," he rationalized. "I'm not going to move twice."

"Oh yes, you are," I snapped. "We cannot keep living together."

"Fine," he snapped back.

Friends of his offered a spare room for free, temporarily. He called it "the closet under the stairs," and Oliver stayed there with him more often than not.

With Roger out of the house, I moved back into our bedroom. My skin crawled to be in that room again. I spent the summer months getting the house ready to list, selling extra furniture on Craigslist, hauling van loads to Goodwill and the dump. Clearing out the house, closets, and storage spaces were heartbreaking work. Toys from the lives of four children, detritus from a family life together. I listed pieces on Craigslist every morning before going to work and arranged to meet buyers after. The weekends were spent digging into the recesses of the house and pulling our history into the light. Roger did not help.

Selling the house was not optional. We couldn't afford the mortgage and rent on a second place. There was, of course, no money. When Roger's free room was no longer available, he moved back home, and it was time for me to move out and list the house. The old place was as ready as I could make it by myself. I had been looking all along for something to rent, anything that would suffice.

Nothing affordable on our side of town was big enough for the kids and me. I was not willing to move away from their schools or into a place with no room for them in hopes that they would come. Marie and Jane were planning to come with me.

I found an affordable three-bedroom apartment in the right area. The cave-like unit would be a gloomy and depressing place to live, but a definite step up from the minivan, which was starting to look like my only other choice. I put in an application and was accepted, a miracle in itself. But, ugh. I asked Jane and Marie if they wanted a dark three bedroom apartment or a nicer two bedroom. They said they would prefer to share a bedroom and live in a less dismal place. I kept looking, frantically now. An advertisement took me to a stretch of road along Bellingham Bay. I hadn't realized there was anything even remotely affordable with a water view. Water views were my favorite rental fantasy.

I drove down State Street as desperate as I've ever felt in my life. I saw the For Rent sign on a shitty building by Boulevard Park, right by the water and pulled in beside the rental agent's car. I followed her around the side of the building and into the unit. The ceilings were low and dingy, and it reeked like an old hotel. There was a bay view, but, oh God, a million years of cigarette smoke permeated the very bones of the place. If I could handle the depression that seemed to come with the apartment like a move-in bonus from hell, I could make it work.

As I was pulling away, application in the passenger's seat, I spotted another For Rent sign two buildings down. A modest place to be sure, but not slummy looking like the first. Somehow, in seventeen years of living in Bellingham, I had never once noticed it.

I called the number immediately. The owner of the building agreed to meet me right away. He led me in, down a long hallway (nice carpet, great paint, no smells) into a spacious living/dining room that overlooked Bellingham Bay in the crystal sunlight. I could practically hear choirs of angels singing. I signed papers on the spot. My deposit check bounced in my brand new single mom account, but I was in.

On my way out of the old house, I scooped up the things I couldn't bear to leave behind: pictures of the kids, a wooden giraffe, a fish-print painting, and a crystal chandelier. My desk and antique farm table. They all fit perfectly into my new space.

I did not have a bed, just our old couch that had become remarkably uncomfortable over the years. The first night, Marie laid on the couch with her head in my lap and cried, missing Jane and Oliver, who had stayed in the house with Roger.

"It's hard to leave your siblings, isn't it?" I asked, stroking her hair.

She nodded into my leg. We stayed there for a long time.

Before the week was over, I found a navy blue loveseat and armchair on Craigslist. The picture was blurry, but I had a feeling about it and went to see. Gorgeous Natuzzi leather, available for a song. The woman selling it was getting divorced. The furniture had sat in her master bedroom unused for years.

"Just like me!" I laughed.

Divorce musical chairs. I also found a like-new mattress set on Craigslist. The seller was kind enough to tie the pieces to the top of my minivan, and I drove it home on Interstate 5 in the rain, hoping the ropes would hold. I hauled that thing into the apartment by myself with minimal damage to it and me and finally had my very own bed.

The first Saturday in the apartment I slept in until 8:00 am. I hadn't had that much sleep in twenty years. I was safe.

Dropping Oliver off at the old house after soccer practice, his body looked small as he stood in the headlights and said, "You don't live here anymore."

"No, I don't," I said.

He turned and went inside. Even now, those words turn my heart to lead. There is no forgiveness for breaking your child's heart. Nor should there be. I desperately wished I could go back and plan a calm separation of some sort without the drama that followed if it would spare my children what they endured. I cannot. I believed that I had done this to them singlehandedly; that I had thoughtlessly wrecked our family with no regard for their pain. Does any parent who gets a divorce ever get over the guilt?

Had I known that my own happiness was a relevant factor in my life; that I was under no obligation to live in misery or mystery... perhaps I would have found the courage to make different choices along the way. The truth is, I willingly gave away my power, looked to Roger to define my life; hid behind my children. I told myself that our struggles weren't any different from those of other people. That our relationship was good and worth keeping. And I decided to stay, over and over, when I should have gone.

The next months were a blur. Marie and I tried to carve out a life together. Jane did not come over much and Oliver, not at all. Alex stayed away. The emotional and financial stress of scraping together enough money for groceries and rent, never quite enough, took its toll. The constant juggling of each child's state of crisis and my own was exhausting. Someone was always falling apart, so I could not. Friends vanished at this point. People don't hang around when you aren't able to buy yourself a beer and pretend like everything is fine. I couldn't care.

Jane turned eighteen and moved in with Marie and me. Oliver still wouldn't come over very often. The old house sold, miraculously. And divorce proceedings were underway. Survival started to seem like a possibility.

During the divorce proceedings, Roger was obligated to turn over his financials and revealed $50,000 in credit card debt, all kept secret from me. I figured his mother would never make him pay back the $43,000 she loaned him, but this was different. All of his accounts but one had already defaulted to collections. There was no protection from these debts for me under the law because the money had been used to support the family, even though I did not know about it. The hope of financial survival dimmed. I sat on my balcony, watching the late afternoon sun glitter on the water, wondering if there was any way I could avoid bankruptcy. *Probably not,* I thought. *Bankruptcy doesn't kill people, though.*

Deep breath. What will come, will come. The sun sank low as a train roared by, yards away.

In addition to working full time at the mental health offices, I began to clean the building on weekends for a few sorely needed extra dollars. Soon after, I took on another office building to clean, and my car payment was made every month, for sure.

The apartment next door connected to mine through a shared laundry room which our neighbor Perry rarely had the opportunity to use. Marie, Jane and I monopolized those appliances with absolute sovereignty. Perry seemed like kind of a weird dude, although it was hard to say why. He did not often leave left his apartment, except to go to Costco, and had a quality that made me want to be careful. Rumor had it he was a day trader. Stories floated around about his confrontations with other neighbors, but he was always civil to me.

One day, he poked his head out of his door as I got home from work.

"Hey, Ronna, come here," he motioned me over.

"Uh, hi, sure," I agreed, surprised at the contact.

I walked to his door, uncertain what he could want.

"I've moved out of my apartment. I'm living in a hotel over on Samish

Way," he divulged.

"Oh, wow, I did not realize that," I responded, surprised. Samish Way was Bellingham's own Skid Row.

"Yeah, I was wondering if you would be willing to help me. I need to get the apartment cleaned out before the end of the month, or those freaking landlords will charge me for another months' rent. Do you know those people have made over $50,000 off of me since I've lived here?"

That's how rent works, I thought. "Oh, umm… sure, I'll help you. What do you need?" I offered.

"Well, before you say yes, take a look inside here. I have a lot of stuff. You can keep or sell anything you find. You should be able to make some money, some of its valuable," he said encouragingly.

"Ok, thanks, Perry. I don't mind helping you out," I said, curious now.

"Well, I want it to be worth it for you. I want you to be able to make some money. Anyway, take a look and tell me what you think. Here are my keys. I'm leaving right now to go back to the hotel. Just text me and let me know." Perry handed me his keyring. "I'm embarrassed at how I've let the place get," he mumbled. "I'm embarrassed for you to see it."

"It's ok, Perry. Don't worry about it," I reassured. "I'll check it out tonight and leave your keys in the mailbox, ok?" I said, turning to open my door.

"NO! Don't do that," Perry sounded alarmed. "Leave the keys over in that planter. There's a plastic bag under the leaves in the dirt."

"Oh, good idea! Will do," I agreed and went inside for dinner, unsure what I had gotten myself into.

After he was gone, I went over to Perry's apartment. Marie and Oliver, who had started coming around, followed me over. I opened the door with his key and slowly entered the dim light of the hall. The air was pungent with the sour stink of smoke and abandonment, and an underlying whiff of filth. A surveillance camera watched from the corner above the door. On closer inspection, I saw that it wasn't connected to anything. The dirty beige carpet of the hall was lined with heavy duty floor mats, the kind used in a mechanic's garage or a warehouse.

We tentatively entered the open door of the first bedroom to the left. There was no furniture. No bed. A narrow pathway wound through piles of boxes and random stuff, as though a load meant for the dump had detoured into the bedroom and flopped on the floor. A broken electric bicycle leaned against the wall. The closet was crammed with ancient, musty men's clothes. I thumbed through the hangers for a minute, wondering if I might find a super valuable classic rock tee shirt. No such luck.

Back in the hall, I pushed open the door to the storage closet off to the right. Some of the built-in shelves were covered with rancid, brown sticky goo. Undeterminable. Other shelves contained rows and rows of bulk-bought Costco cleaning supplies. I would never have to buy toilet bowl cleaner or Lysol again. A shop vac and upright vacuum cleaner stood in the corner. So far, so good for value.

Marie and Oliver tiptoed ahead of me into the second bedroom. Teetering towers of empty Amazon boxes left just enough room to squeeze the door open. The room was impassable; any light from the window was obscured by the stacks, which began to topple, packaging bubbles floating to the floor.

"I can't even get to the light switch," Oliver grunted, trying reach behind a stack without knocking it over.

"If we were gonna find bodies, they're gonna be in here," Marie whispered.

As Marie stepped into the room, her foot came down on an air pillow packing bubble from one of the Amazon boxes, which popped with a bang, as if from a gunshot. The kids screamed and dissolved into nervous giggles. I peered past their heads into the room at the rows of silver shelving racks lined with plastic storage bins that filled the room. The back wall was impossible to see, but those shelving units were worth something.

Marie is right, God knows what we're going to find in this room, I thought. *There could definitely be bodies.*

Back across the hall, the bathroom, beyond filthy, had apparently never been cleaned. The outside of the toilet was a mass of pubic hair stuck to grime, dust, and pee. The inside of the bowl was slightly cleaner, just mold and the requisite ring. The bathtub was covered with a layer of pink slime.

"I hope there are some rubber gloves in all those cleaning supplies," I said with a grimace as the kids made puking noises and hurried toward the living room. While they continued to explore, I entered the kitchen.

"Mom, Mom," Marie shouted from the living room. "This peanut tin is full of MONEY!" she yelled, rattling a clinking container.

"Cool! Keep it!" I called from the kitchen. "If you'll help, you can keep all the change you find."

"SWEET!" she said as she began ripping lids off the peanut tins that lined another shelving unit. Some tins were full of change, and some had empty capsule parts, tiny baggies, and plastic droppers.

The kitchen countertops were solid sheets of stickiness. I tried to pick up a blender, an expensive one, but it was glued to the counter in a ring of that brown goo. I tried to move other appliances, utensils, anything laying on the counter. Everything was stuck. The cupboards were full of filthy, high-end cookware, all of it melted and wrecked. I inched around the backside of the walk-through kitchen, between filing cabinets and a table piled with papers, and into the living room. A 52-inch big screen television covered one window, blocking the view of Bellingham Bay. Banks of computers with slick monitors sat on a Geek desk. More shelving units piled with boxes and peanut tins formed a barricade around the computer and TV area, the singular open space in the entire apartment. This was where Perry hung out.

"This desk is SO COOL," Oliver exclaimed, pushing the buttons that raised and lowered it. "Look at all these cases of Monster drinks under here! Can I have them?"

"You can have one pack," I allowed. "That much Monster would kill you."

"Aww, Mommm," he complained, but quickly forgot as Marie pulled a half gallon jar of personal lube out of a cardboard box.

"AAHHHH," she yelled, dropping it back in.

"Oh my God," I moaned. "Sweetie, just go wash your hands, ok?"

She ran back to our apartment through the laundry room to scrub, taking her peanut tins full of money.

Perry's computers, monitors, desk, and television had to be worth several thousand dollars. I googled GEEK desk. Yep, big bucks. There could be more valuable items tucked away in the scary second bedroom. I needed the money, and I knew exactly how to tackle this project. I had been here before.

"When do you want me to start?" I texted Perry.

I got started the next night as soon as I got home from work. I cleaned Perry's apartment every night after work and all weekend every weekend, carving out time to go back to the offices to clean those, too. It took me a solid month to clear the place out.

Inside the storage containers on the shelving racks in the scary second bedroom, we found immaculate and painstakingly stored cans and jars. Recycling. Perry had washed and stored his recycling in sturdy plastic bins with flip-top lids. His recycling was worthless, but the bins were not. Behind the plastic bins were shelves of tools. Nice tools. Hundreds of dollars' worth of tools. And a six foot tall red Craftsman tool cabinet on wheels, which had not been visible from the bedroom door. Consider how full a small bedroom must be to completely obscure a 6 foot tall, bright red cabinet. Fishing rods. Stacks of wooden cigar boxes, most still full of cigars. The cigars had been improperly stored and were unwrapped, rolling around loose in the boxes. I sold them anyway. A newspaper with a headline of JFK's murder from Perry's hometown was stuffed in the bottom of a toolbox. And more clothes, old suits, and yellowed dress shirts.

Craigslist took care of the tools and red cabinet, floor mats, electric bike, shelving units, shop vac, furniture, and cigars. The recycling filled the can by the street, with plenty left over for the following weeks. Once the recycling had been taken out, I sold the plastic storage bins on Craigslist, too. The JFK newspaper went to the library. Garbage bag after garbage bag went to the dump, the cans by the street long since stuffed. Marie and Oliver helped, squealing every time they stepped into the second bedroom and set off a BANG of bubble wrap, hauling their treasures through the laundry room to our apartment.

The gigantic TV went to my living room, where it still sits, the Geek desk and computer went to Oliver's bedroom at his dad's house. Marie kept all the loose change, which turned out to be several hundred dollars. Several years went by before I had to buy cleaning supplies. To this day, I have giant rolls of aluminum foil and saran wrap and one fantastic omelet pan.

After every garbage bag was gone and every surface scrubbed, I left the keys for the landlord. Last I heard, Perry had landed in Thailand to teach English. He emailed a picture of himself in a classroom with a thatch roof, surrounded by smiling young women. He looked delighted. I had made at least a thousand extra bucks and shared an adventure with my kids that we still laugh about.

A month or so later, my three oldest kids met at the apartment without Oliver, for a difficult conversation. Roger was not hiding his online activities from the kids, which made them uncomfortable. They needed it to stop. We discussed how to approach the situation.

While we talked, I texted Roger and gave him an ultimatum: I would call CPS unless he ceased all sexual activity when the kids were in the house and kept his computer in his room. He was furious. They will never know the viciousness of the exchange that took place while they huddled on my living room floor. Jane texted her grandmother to enlist her help. Roger would listen to his mother.

The kids came to the conclusion that an intervention was in order. They would sit down with Roger asking for a change in his behavior. If he were unwilling to agree, they would move in with me. At the time, Marie and Oliver were living with Roger in his three-bedroom rental house, while Jane stayed with me. Alex lived with college friends. Our separate homes had developed revolving doors with kids moving freely back and forth depending on their current moods and who they were most angry at on any given day.

As the kids made arrangements for their meeting, I began to prepare to move to a bigger place. My current lease still had six months to go so I would have to find someone to sublet the apartment and find money for a deposit on a new one. My first thought was to go back to the apartment complex where I had initially found a three bedroom unit. None were available. Back to Craigslist. What did people do before Craigslist?

Two nights later, while the kids sat down with their father, I visited a reasonably priced three bedroom duplex a couple of streets away. The place looked like a trash heap made of particle board on the outside, but the inside was lovely and clean with gleaming hardwood floors, a fenced yard for Brutus, the Yorkie-poo, and a sparkling kitchen. The third bedroom was technically a closet with just enough room to turn around, but I did not care. Marie and Oliver could have the real bedrooms. Jane could share with Marie or, more likely, move in with her college friends. If the planets aligned and I could come up with money for the deposit and simultaneously find someone to sublet my apartment, I could make it happen. I did not see how these pieces could fall into place before the end of the week. But they had to.

While the kids were at Roger's, I drove home in sheer panic as I mulled over ways to pull this move together. Nothing was coming to mind. If I defaulted on my current lease, the landlords would surely come after me for the money. I could not ask my mother for a deposit. She had sent grocery money several times over the last year, even though I never asked. I was grateful for her help, but I could not ask her for more. This was a sobering reality. The stakes were high. I had to find a way. Despair rose like buzzing bees, and I felt my tenuous grip of control starting to slip in earnest. I made it home and went straight to the balcony.

Jane came home and sat down beside me. Roger had listened. He moved his computer into his bedroom and agreed to hide his activities from Marie and Oliver. They decided to stay with him, and I did not have to move. They were giving him one more chance. Jane would stay with me. My panic subsided. I stayed on the deck watching the movement of the water, relief moving through my body like the light on the waves. We would be okay for now, until the next hit. Long lost lyrics from an old hymn trailed through my head... *like a tree standing by the water, I shall not be moved.*

Arkansas

Time in Arkansas was an intermission from the day to day of my soul-scraping childhood. There was Grandpa. There was Uncle Bill. There was Berryville and Oak Grove. Rolling green hills, junior rodeos with greased pigs, and the rank smell of chicken farms. We went in the summer sometimes, to see family. There was still church, but it was a little country church where everyone was related. There was Grandma and Grandpa's house, hanging out on the big covered front porch watching pickup trucks chug by on the dusty road out front, and sleeping in the loft with the drop-down ladder.

Behind the house, we clambered through morning glory vines over the top of the underground cellar. When tornado warnings came on the radio, and the sky turned green, we hid in that spider-ridden darkness, sitting in between shelves of Grandma's jars of canned apricots and green beans. A rope swing hung from the old walnut tree by the gate that led to the pasture and barn, where we couldn't go alone because Grandpa's horse, Rusty, kicked. Grandpa chopped the heads off chickens, headless bodies flapped across the grass, still squawking, while their heads lay in a pile beside the chopping stump. Grandma held the bodies upside down over the big sink in the utility room grimly stripping feathers off.

On the other side of the yard was Grandma's garden, rows and rows of vegetables to be avoided in case there was a call to weed. Raspberry vines grew on the fence, and Concord grapes twined the wire, juicy tang bursting in my mouth, as I chased fireflies in the dusk.

My cousins and sisters and I ran through the gravelly dirt beside the road to the intersection that was the town of Oak Grove. The wood framed screen door to the only store in town banged, springless, as we selected grape Crush and Kool candy cigarettes. We guzzled soda and pretended to smoke on a slow walk home.

Every kid should have a fun uncle, the one who takes time to hang out and jokes around. Uncle Bill was that guy, and I adored him. His two front teeth were a bridge that he could pop out with his tongue, to great effect. I howled every time and begged him to do it again. Uncle Bill came from a family of big Ozark people in overalls who lived in Berryville, or around. They were hysterically funny, and quick-witted, and so warm and kind. I had never met anyone like them; still haven't, I guess.

Sometimes we got to go swimming in the creek with Uncle Bill and the cousins. Crystal clear, sun-warmed water rippled over smooth stones at the bank, the stream ever cooler toward the middle, where I couldn't touch. The deep part under the bridge was called Devil's Hole. Some of the kids were brave enough to jump off, but I wasn't. My sisters and I could wear swimsuits in front of family, so we did not have to swim in dresses.

Uncle Bill took me out to the middle of the creek to paddle around, and when I had to go to the bathroom, he said, "Go ahead!"

"In the water?" I shrieked with delight and started to pee.

"Swim away, swim away," he yelled, laughing. "You gotta go downstream! Now swish around to get rid of the warm spot." He cracked up as I twisted and churned, then grabbed my hand and pulled me back. Creek etiquette.

Even though he had been raped multiple times by a Pentecostal preacher as a young child, Uncle Bill believed. He believed in God. He believed in love. He believed in humor. No bitterness lived in him. Yesterday, I found a letter he wrote to me.

I now realize what the Arkansas experience meant to you. How little did I know of the constraints of trying to live your life in a box. Around us, you were able to be what you wanted without worrying if someone was watching or whether your actions would be reported to the judges (and there were many) who sat on their thrones of self-exaltation and reported all infractions of the rules to the political elite. What a sham! If anything I gave you has contributed to the beautiful person that you are, then I am deeply touched and humbled. We never know what our lives are saying to others. That's why it's so important to be real and to always reach out to all who cross our paths.

Years later, not long before Uncle Bill died, I went to see him. I had disassociated from my family for a time, including from him. In my bitterness and avoidance, I shunned his attempts to reach out, afraid he would tell me to go to church, to return to the fold. No one wants to be pressured to return to their abuser with open arms. I felt I had to protect myself at all costs, even from him. We took a slow walk around the block on that last visit. Then I sat beside him in his recliner for a while, his arms wrapped tightly around me.

I am grateful for these memories.

Chapter 17
Refuge

I gaze at the wide stone staircase of the Sacre-Couer cathedral that stretches up the hillside in front of me. Towering white walls gleam in the summer sun, light bounces off curvaceous domes braced against the brilliant blue Parisian sky. The Sacre-Couer is unlike every other cathedral I have visited, with soft architecture and rounded spires reminiscent of the Mediterranean. This cathedral has none of the aggressive gothic spikes and dark monstrosity of the others, which have all been sharp edges and spines, weapons and gargoyles; pain and oppression plastered to every surface. Fear guarded every door, but this church is different.

July heat soaks into my body as I climb the staircase toward the Sacre-Coeur's open doors. I step onto the terrace at the top and turn around. Paris spreads out as far as I can see, flat and dull in the summer haze, the Eiffel Tower just visible through the trees. I am really here. I am traveling through Europe with my new love; divorce four years in the past; no longer a fresh wound.

I follow the flow of tourists into the cool shade of the chapel, immediately enveloped in peaceful, hushed quiet. Sunlight filters softly through the high windows casting an otherworldly sheen to the air. Walls swoop up to a concave frescoed ceiling, all light, soft curves, and love. *This cathedral seems female*, I think. Unlike the dark judgmental penetrative spikes of the others and the suffocating oppression of the churches of my childhood. I can breathe here.

I walk the perimeter of the nave to a candle stand and clink my euros into the tin box. I select four white tea candles, one for each of my children, and place them on the stand. As I light the candles one by one, I bring each child to mind and whisper words of prayer for their protection, as I have done at every cathedral visit. It can't hurt to ask, just in case someone is listening. Solace comes in hope; the feel of the candles' soft wax, the flicker of flame as one wick touches the next, the act of asking for mercy on behalf of another. I remember words of advice I have come to live by, grace I was given.

"Here's the thing, Ronna, the way to get your kids through this time," Gary said to me when my divorce was new, his voice low and serious. "You gotta do the right thing every day as best you can. Do what you know is right, and it will pay off." My sister, Karissa, and her husband were visiting. We sat on my balcony with full glasses of better cabernet than I could afford.

Gary leaned forward, his white hair gleaming in the fading light as the sun sank into the bay and color flooded the sky, blue to turquoise, pink and orange. "Just take it one day at a time, sometimes hour by hour, even moment by moment. Take a deep breath and stick with it."

"Eventually, the kids will see it," he reassured as the light faded to black. Stars blinked on. I hoped he was right. I knew perseverance was my only option, anyway.

Being a parent my kids can depend on, taking care of them any way I can, the best that I can, is its own reward. Working as hard as possible for as many hours a day as possible never feels like enough-not enough money, not enough effort, no way to make up for what has been lost. My children will never know the gut-wrenching heartache of my failures. But they come around, tease me, invade my kitchen and sprawl on my carpet, monopolize my remote control, show up unannounced for dinner, and love me. Their presence is everything.

During those dark days after the divorce, some days were hell. A lot of days were hell. Gary will never know how many times I chanted his advice to myself like a prayer. One foot in front of the other, one breath at a time, stop and listen. Repeat. My escape was to never miss a sunset if I could help it. In the process, my sharp edges began to soften, the chainsaw buzz in my head slowed to a hum, and I was able to see the beauty in front of me.

I spent as much time as I could carve out of any given day sitting on my balcony. Early morning runs on the boardwalk, through mist and pre-dawn light before the day begins, and then rush straight home after work whenever possible to sit with the bay. Under starlight, blazing sun, misty mornings and surreal, fiery sunsets, I have watched the sky and water. I have watched the sunset move across the horizon with the seasons, watched snow fall on the water, geese skim the surface, loons dive, and seagulls careen and stalk my deck for bits of barbecue. Herons glide, seals bob and boats come and go. I have watched the Coast Guard, helicopter training exercises, barges, sailboat races, fishing boats, kayaks, and canoes. Never the same scene twice.

The soft stillness of the Sacre-Couer envelopes me like those sunsets, shining through the cracks of my soul, seeping into the last dark corners of fear, the not knowing, the guilt, all laid bare. I wander around to the other side of the sanctuary, not glancing at the statues and historical plaques, through the roped entrance to the rows of wooden pews, and slide into a seat. Leaning back, I study the fresco of Jesus that soars above, painted in gold and white and soft blues. His arms outstretched, his face benign. An elderly woman to my right catches my attention. She crosses herself by a statue of Mary; her movements have the careless grace of habit. I watch as she kisses her fingertips and touches them to Mary's stone toes.

Perhaps I just witnessed a mother to mother prayer because the mother of Jesus would understand. Perhaps she is passing her worries out of her body. I wonder how many mothers have left cares on those cold, stone toes. Mothers of warriors, of children lost or sick or sad, grief for their own fears and failures and helplessness. We must release it all somewhere or go mad. I remember my own solitary walks to work through the woods and down to the sea during the disintegration of my marriage. Movement and silence cleared my mind for the deluge of the day to come and from the chaos at home. I thought of my own mother, whose unshakeable faith anchored her through the traumas that came her way.

A few months before, I visited Mom for the weekend. We shopped, went out for dinner and played Scrabble, which I lost, as always. She remains unbeatable. Afterward, we settled onto the couch with cups of tea for the usual chats about family gossip.

Mom leaned toward me, peered at me over the top of her glasses.

"Do you believe in God at all?" she asked, her gray eyes held a glint of challenge that matched her tone.

Her question took me by surprise, but I knew what she meant. She meant do you believe in God the way I taught you to; do you believe in MY God, her

God of rigid rules, judgment and the straight and narrow way. She raised me up in the way I should go with the Biblical promise that I would not depart from it. But I did. I never could resist a meandering trail.

"No, Mom, I don't," I replied honestly. Her religion, which laid waste to my God-given autonomy, holds no power over me now. What's mine is mine, and what's mine is me.

She lowered her gaze in silence, shoulders slumped with disappointment, my rejection personal. She believes I am going to Hell. This makes her sad, and I am sad for her. She cannot join me in a conversation about different renditions of belief, or express curiosity about my interpretation of the divine. I cannot expect her to. This single question is as far as she will go. Unwilling to explain or defend, I will not move closer to her, either, a silent truce called.

I can admit Roger broke my heart when he turned away from me. He broke my heart with his secret. But my heart was in a million pieces long before I met Roger, I simply laid it at his feet and said step here. I expected him to fix my brokenness for me.

As my fatigue and anger subside, I have found the freedom to sort through my dismantled self. I created a home of my own, a place to remember who I am; an island where I fell in love with my own life. When my children are here, they feel at home. Not because they grew up in these walls or have childhood memories of it, but because this is the place their mother became real. They come and go and come back again, returning to me like waves on the rocks. Sometimes I find evidence of their hanging out. Stray socks and water glasses, hairbands, and joints. They come here and hide, bring friends, talk to me all night, or be sick and sleep in my bed, eat all of my food, complain that there is no food. And they sit by the water and watch.

As I sit in the cathedral, pieces of me arrive on waves of light. I steady myself as they return to their rightful places. A melting sensation spreads through my chest, and my heart begins to weep. I rest my arms on the bench in front of me and breathe deeply to avoid having to explain my tears to my lover, which I do not want to do. If I had it to do over again, I would let those tears fall like rain.

Later that night, seated on the still sun-warmed steps of the Sacre-Couer, the bright white full summer moon rises and hangs over Paris like the spotlight of the world. Groups of young people cluster on the terraced steps, singing, drinking, smoking, laughing; bathing in the moonlight. Deep velvet air surrounds us all. My future husband wraps his arm around my waist and kisses me, and when the stone steps grow cold, leads me to our bed, to his arms.

I remember now, who I was in the first place. That girl before she became afraid; before she learned to subvert and hide. The day will come when I say goodbye to my balcony by the water, the place that saved my soul, healed my heart and, sunset by sunset pieced me back together. I will trust love while knowing sometimes it fails. Or maybe it doesn't. Perhaps love exists like currents in the sea if only we can fall into the stream. What comes next is a new adventure and love and the next big thing. I'll never be fully prepared, but I am comfortable with that uncertainty.

I'm almost ready.

Epilogue

Just relax the voice inside my head barks.

I **am** *relaxed*, I snap back.

I mean, I'm trying. It's harder than you think, I whine to myself.

I held my breath, standing on the brink of something.

Shut out of something.

Stumbling in the dark, I scraped against a crack in the wall, saw a narrow band of light streaming through.

Oh, it's here, my insides screamed.

Then beating sobbing fighting pushing pulling and punching my way out with a splintering crash.

I am breathing hard and am somewhat bloodied.

Now what? I ask the open air with fists still clenched.

I'm here, he said.

What if I disappoint you? I wondered to myself but only nodded as he gently unfolded my fingers.

A lucky thing to not have missed love when it arrived. To hold its beating heart in my open hand and stroke the soft down. It is quite another to expose the untended corners of my own heart, to stop trying to figure out who and how to be and just be.

Can I let you in, all the way in, where the sour bits desiccate, the dark heart places that have never seen light? Can I let you accept my failures?

Can I let you love me anyway?

He said one time, he said *if it doesn't work out in the end, it's been wonderful.*

And my heart sank because my head pounded with the need for a guarantee, but it turns out that's not what love is. Love is not a contract or a deadline or an ultimatum or a deal or even a safety net. And then my heart rose because he loved me enough to not lie.

As it turns out, love is a whisper in the night, a *how was your day*, a pat on the hip that means something more and listening without waiting for a turn. Love is making the effort, wanting to. Love is always turning toward.

And the ravishing.

It's all here.

So, relax. Just relax.

About the Author

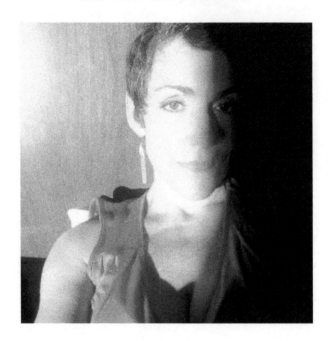

Ronna Russell grew up the youngest daughter of a well-known United Pentecostal preacher. From an early age, Ronna plotted to escape the church, hell or no hell. She jumped into marriage at the age of twenty-three, a union that lasted 22 years and produced four children. When the marriage ended, Ronna found herself free to consider her own desires. With these transitions behind her and her children grown, Ronna has relocated, remarried and returned to school.

Thank you so much for reading one of our **Biography / Memoirs**.
If you enjoyed our book, please check out our recommended title for your next great read!

Z.O.S. by Kay Merkel Boruff

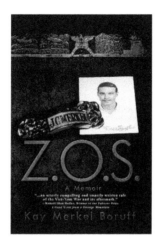

"...dazzling in its specificity and intensity."

–C.W. Smith, author of *Understanding Women*

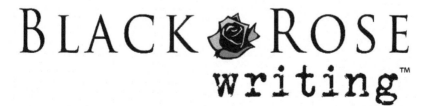

CPSIA information can be obtained
at www.ICGtesting.com
Printed in the USA
LVHW041707281119
638727LV00021B/2374/P

9 781684 332373